DIAGNOSIS: HIV SERIES

HIV and Me

Firsthand Information for Coping with HIV and AIDS

By Timothy Critzer

Firsthand Books • San Francisco, California

© Copyright 2004, Timothy Critzer

Firsthand Books
584 Castro Street #342
San Francisco, CA 94114
www.FirsthandBooks.com

Publishers Cataloging-in-Publication Data

Critzer, Timothy.
    HIV and me : firsthand information for coping with HIV and AIDS / by Timothy Critzer. 1st ed. San Francisco, Calif. : Firsthand Books, 2004.

        p. cm.
        (Diagnosis: HIV series)
        Includes bibliographical references.
        ISBN: 0-9745388-3-3

        1. HIV infections--Psychological aspects. 2. HIV-positive persons.
    3. HIV infections. 4. AIDS (Disease) Psychological aspects.
    5. AIDS (Disease) Patients. 6. AIDS (Disease) I. Title.

RC606.64 .C75 2004   2004092224
362.196/9792--dc22   0406

Editor: Paul M. Howey
Cover Design: George Foster
Composition: Kristen Butler
Printed in the United States of America

What people are saying about this book . . .

"This tool is a great resource for the newly diagnosed or people that haven't been able to come to terms with the fact that they are HIV-positive. The book is easy to understand, and the exercise instructions are very easy to follow."

Brenda Kreiger, RN
Matthew 25 AIDS Services

"'HIV and Me' brings clarity to the many complex and challenging issues surrounding living with HIV. Timothy Critzer has a richly engaging writing style that readers will enjoy. He has written a book that I wish had been around when I received my HIV diagnosis. . . . I learned many things that will help me in my day-to-day life. . . ."

Paul Serchia
Formerly of AIDS Project Los Angeles

"'HIV and Me' is a blessing. It is a roadmap on a journey to living in peace for persons with HIV and AIDS. It is very well written, clear and to the point, and should be given to everyone . . . with HIV or AIDS as a companion for peaceful living. It is necessary to be read by health and social service professionals who will find it helpful in assisting persons with these conditions, as well as reminding us how our [clients] evolve on the journey toward peace with their illness."

Annette Horvath, MS, HSA
Ray Riordan, CSW
Village Care of New York

"The author's personal sharing contained in the book is powerful and sincere. He provides practical advice and guidance to successfully navigate the emotional, bureaucratic and medical challenges people face. The book consistently reinforces the need for someone to move ahead at their pace and in their time. The tone of the writing is deeply personal, sensitive and nurturing. He addresses consumer reactions and concerns directly and honestly. I highly recommend the book for consumers, volunteers and professionals. We all have an opportunity to learn a great deal from this publication."

Kevin J. Burns, LCSW, QCSW
Action AIDS

"'HIV and Me' is a wonderful tool for someone newly diagnosed with HIV. It guides the reader in thinking through complex issues in an interactive format that may prove invaluable for bringing a sense of order to a time that is often hallmarked by overwhelm. . . . Unlike many workbooks that people complete and leave, this one will likely prove a resource for an individual to return to time and again as their thinking and experiences change overtime."

Brenda Lein
Project Inform

"I would like to say that, having worked as a caregiver and psychotherapist and educational trainer for people with HIV since 1984, I find this work very approachable and accessible, especially for people who may not know "where to start" in their process of putting HIV in its proper perspective. I really like the consistent return to the concept of "balance" throughout the writing. It is a concept which helps to reduce anxiety and in particular the need to be "the perfect HIV patient", which is such a huge issue for so many people."

Alan J. Brown, PHD, MFT
The L.I.F.E. Program

"As a long-time nurse and counselor in the HIV/AIDS community, I welcome this book, which can really be of benefit for many of my patients who are dealing with the issues of life after a HIV diagnosis. I think that, regardless of gender or social status, the human issues of self-worth, mortality and survival are universal, and I would gladly give this book to all my patients. Its lesson of recovering from crisis and reformulating life is something all my [clients] could benefit from. I highly recommend this book for all HIV practices."

Eileen Wall, RN, MFT-R
Counselor

Contents

Acknowledgments

I would like to thank Sue Rose, Carl Mullen and Jim Beitzel for being my cheerleaders, encouraging me to bring my vision into reality.

I would like to thank those people that shared their expertise and experience to ensure that readers receive meaningful, accurate information upon which to base their decisions.

I would like to thank those people that reviewed my manuscript and helped me to bring the best guidance possible to those whom need it the most right now, especially David Armagnac, Clare Connors and Michael Mancilla.

I would like to thank George Foster for the polish, professionalism and perseverance he exhibited in getting just the right cover that matched the feeling of this book.

I would like to thank Crisanta Johnson, Becky Kelleher, Nadine Burg, James Goldstein and Jeff Snowden for being my support network, without which I would have had a difficult time reaching my place of peace with HIV.

I would like to thank Lisa Talamantez for being the best cosmic sibling that a person could ever hope for.

Finally, I would like to thank my family for accepting my HIV status without hesitation, an act that enabled me to find my peace with HIV much more quickly.

Disclaimer

The statements and opinions in this book are not meant to replace the advice or treatment of a therapist, counselor, physician or other licensed caregiver. The reader is encouraged to seek out those resources as needed in their own situation. The inclusion of publications and websites in this book is for the purpose of providing the reader with a sample of available resources, not as an endorsement of any nature of those individual publications or websites listed. The resource lists provided are a sample of those available and are by no means exhaustive. I encourage each reader to seek out additional resources as needed within their own situation. Any description of my use of a product is not intended to be an endorsement of that product for use by anyone other than myself. I encourage each reader to make his or her own independent evaluation of any product mentioned within this book. I have no commercial or financial affiliation with any of the manufacturers, wholesalers or retailers of these products.

All of the information about websites, publications and medical studies is current as of the writing of this book. However, HIV and its treatments are constantly changing, so some information within this book may be out of date by the time this book is published. The reader is encouraged to do his or her own research and verification of said information before relying upon any of it. If you do find that something has significantly changed, please let me know by email at *Timothy@HIVandMe.com* so that I can include this important new information in future editions. My goal is to continue to provide the most accurate information to everyone that needs that helping hand in learning how to live in peace with HIV and AIDS.

Preface

Before I help you to begin your journey, I'd like to tell you who I am, who I'm not and why I was moved to write this book. I think it is important that you know all three of these things if the information within this book is going to help you to find your peace.

My name is Timothy Critzer, and I am HIV-positive. During the five years since my diagnosis in October 1998, I have taken an incredible journey in my HIV life. This path I followed had caused me to travel through some of the darkest places that the human spirit can find, places that I stayed in for years. It was only when I finally realized that my life was worth saving that I found my peace with HIV and AIDS, emerging into the light to begin living my life again. Once this peace took hold in my life, I realized that I needed to share with other HIV-positive people my experiences along this journey and the wisdom gained from them. I felt like I had discovered a secret formula for how to live a full life with HIV in it, and I wanted to find a way to help as many people as possible to do the same. My goal was and still is for every HIV-positive person to experience this renewed sense of being alive, this important recognition that their life is not damaged or ruined and this sense of peace and acceptance about having HIV and AIDS in their life, instead of the common panic and fear it brings.

All that being said, one question likely still comes to your mind—why should you take advice from me on this topic? Good question. And it deserves a good answer. Besides the knowledge and experience from my own journey, I have education, training and experience in law, accounting, human resources, insurance, benefits, nutrition, fitness, healing, holistic medicine, counseling, and communication. Also, I have volunteered or worked at many different types of HIV/AIDS service organizations, while at the same time also using their services as a HIV-positive client. Along the way, I've meet thousands of people that are trying to learn to live with HIV and AIDS, and many of them have shared with me their thoughts, feelings and experiences. Their experiences and mine are part of a tribal wisdom that people with HIV and AIDS have created as a result of living with these conditions. So it turns out that I hadn't discovered any secret formula about how to live peacefully with HIV; instead, I had uncovered a body of knowledge about this topic that exists in the lives of people already doing it. It is this tribal wisdom, along with my own education and training, that I have documented and used to create a roadmap for you in this book. This roadmap is meant to help you chart your own course towards living in peace with HIV and AIDS, using other people's insight and guidance for support. So even though I have used my own life as an example to guide you, the materials in this book are designed to help *you* create a plan of action that fits *your* own life, your own unique experience with HIV.

Before you begin reading this book, it is important that you understand that I am not a licensed therapist or a physician. I am also not a lawyer or a licensed social worker. My words and advice in this book should not be used as a substitute for the care, treatment or services of these and other highly skilled professionals, whenever you need it in your life. Learning to take advantage of all the resources available to support your new life with HIV is one of the keys to finding that peace I have spoken of. However, that being said, I do want you to know that several licensed professionals that work in the HIV/AIDS field have reviewed this book's material. Each of these professionals has recognized the book as a valuable tool for helping people to deal with their HIV diagnosis in a real life way, as evidenced by their comments in the opening pages of this book. Also, HIV/AIDS service organizations across the country have put the book to use in assisting their clients to get out of crisis and to begin living their lives again after diagnosis. So when I tell you that I *truly* believe that what the book contains can help you to find that peace with HIV in your own life, I'm doing so with added confidence of knowing that these highly skilled HIV professionals believe it too.

As a resource for your journey, I've created a website, *www.HIVandMe.com*, where you can find updates to information in this book and links to other sites that might be helpful as you move along your path. If you visit the site and have comments or suggestions, I encourage you to share them with me by emailing me from the link on the site. Also, be sure to check this site for news and updates on future projects of mine that may be helpful to you, like workshops, seminars and new publications.

Now that I've done what I can to get you started, the rest is up to you. Only you can do the emotional and mental work to get past the news of your diagnosis and on with the business of living. Only you can work through the exercises in this book and create a plan of action to deal with how HIV affects your every day life. Only you can decide that your life is still worth living, no matter what happens in it. Only you.

Timothy

Foreword
By Michael Mancilla, MSW, LICSW

Papaya enzymes. Bitter melons. Chinese herbs and acupuncture. These were what composed my grocery list of things that I had to have if I was going to survive and thrive with this illness. While I may still have a dusty bottle of papaya enzymes somewhere in my attic, I could not begin to recall what it was for; all I do know is that eleven years later, I am surviving without it.

Surviving is what Timothy Critzer brings our attention to in his second book, *HIV and Me*. Combining practical suggestions with a self-assured level of insight that comes from living with this disease, he shares what has worked for him, and more importantly, what may work for you.

Underlying his writing and guided journal exercises is a subtle spirituality that frames both his own experiences and his common sense advice. Critzer brings his own voice as an openly HIV+ man into the new world of living with this illness, a world where death is a bit more elusive and the challenges we face perhaps more varied. The confidence and empathy he brings to issues such as disclosure, medications, and legal matters create a feeling that you have a trusted friend, someone who can act as a touchstone as you begin to make sense of it all.

Voices such as Critzer's are sadly less heard from today. Ask yourself, do we live more "normal" lives now as people with HIV? In doing so, are we given the luxury to struggle more quietly than our predecessors, who engaged in protests and die-ins during the heydays of ACT-UP and red-ribbon celebrity events? Answering this, the author heralds us into a new era as people living with HIV, in that he fulfills a need to speak with authority and authenticity. As such, he continues in the footsteps of Jesse Jackson, who once said "You cannot teach what you don't know. You cannot give energy if you're not on fire on the inside"

Turn the page and begin to walk across the embers.

Michael Mancilla MSW, LICSW
Co-author *Love in The Time of HIV:*
The Gay Man's Guide to Sex,
Dating and Relationships

*To Carl and David,
and the thousands of others like them
who have learned to live in peace with
HIV and AIDS*

Introduction

The Journey Towards Peace
Starts Now

It was probably the most shocking news of your life. Maybe you already knew on some level, or perhaps it was a complete surprise. Either way, once your fear of catching HIV is confirmed as a reality, shock is what sets in. I learned this first-hand on October 6, 1998, the day that I was told that I am HIV-positive. I went completely numb. I had suspected that something was wrong with my health since May of that year when I had the worst flu of my life. It left me feeling too weak to stand, which no illness had ever done. Six weeks later, half the hair on my head fell out. I freaked out. Luckily, it all grew back. A month later, I developed tiny painful sores in my mouth during a period of extreme stress. The evidence was mounting that something had drastically changed within my health, though it still took me two more months to summon up enough courage to take an HIV test. Suspecting the worst, I used a mail-in home test where you phone in for the results, just so I wouldn't have to face the sympathetic look of a test counselor if they told me that I had HIV. Suspicion confirmed. HIV present. Let the crisis begin.

Crisis is likely the best way to describe your state right now. You may be asking yourself, "Why did this have to happen to me?" You might be imagining all sorts of horrible stuff for your future, and maybe even hoping that you will wake up from this nightmare at any second. If you are anything like me, you are also wishing that someone would tell you how to deal with this news, how to stop HIV from ruining your life and what to do to have the best chance for a long, happy future. Wish granted. Using this book, I plan to conceptually take you by the shoulder, sit you gently in a chair and fill your head, heart and life with the firsthand wisdom and guidance necessary for you to move from your crisis to living in peace with HIV. Living in peace with HIV? Maybe this is tough for you to imagine at this point, but I and thousands of others with HIV have found that peace in our daily lives. I am certain that you will too.

This book is organized to follow your likely path on this journey, one from crisis to acceptance to peace. Your journey is divided into four stages: *Ending Your Crisis, Building Your Foundation, Managing Your Details* and *Achieving Your Balance. Ending Your Crisis* in Chapter 1 is designed to help you take control of your mind and end your current crisis state. *Building Your Foundation* in Chapters 2 through 4 is meant to show you how to put a solid foundation under your journey. Once you have become more centered and grounded, *Managing Your Details* in Chapters 5 and 6 is ready to assist you in contemplating daily life issues that may arise as a result of your new status. *Achieving Your Balance* in Chapter 7 will help you to find the balance between mind, body and spirit in your life, a state that should lead you to vibrant health and happiness. It is important that you read the chapters in this book in the order in which they are presented. Each new stage builds upon what you have learned in the last one. Therefore, you won't get any benefit from moving to the next stage until after you have mastered the topics and techniques of the current stage. I know that you probably want to finish the whole book now, thinking that that will get you to a place of peace. Unfortunately, the process is not that easy. The peace that you seek will only come in its own time, not when you try and force it. Skipping ahead in the process will only serve to overwhelm you and cause you stress, anxiety, and discomfort as you contemplate subjects that you don't yet have the foundation to handle. Take it from someone that knows.

There is no timeline for your journey towards peace, and no need for you to rush its completion. You will get there when you get there. You may feel like you are racing against time, but you are not. I can tell you that you won't complete your journey in a day, a week or a month. It may take months for you to finish one stage, or as in my case, maybe years. Unlike me, though, you have the benefit of this book to guide you, so your journey may be swifter than mine. It all depends upon how much effort that you put into it. Refer to this book often to reaffirm what you have learned as you work through each area of your life affected by HIV. Just take it one step at a time, go at your own speed and create the lasting peace that you are seeking.

I have followed up the discussion in each chapter with helpful exercises for each topic covered. Using a notebook as your journal, you can create a strategy that fits your life for dealing with each topic. Here is how it works: the discussion portion brings a topic into your mind and starts you thinking, and then the exercises focus you on putting your thoughts down on paper and working through them to come up with a plan of action for that topic. This complete process may help you master each stage of your journey more easily, allowing you to adjust to your new status more quickly. Use the checklist at the end of each chapter to determine if you have completed all the work necessary for you to take the next step in your journey.

After the exercises in each chapter, you will find a list of resources that relate to that chapter's topics. These lists are meant to give you an idea of the types of resources available to assist you. They are best used as a starting point for you to go out on your own and find more resources to support the transition that you are now experiencing.

Don't forget to jot down in your journal any immediate thoughts that you may have while reading. Sometimes those thoughts that just pop into your head are the most valuable information for your healing. Be sure to get them down in your journal before they disappear. In fact, I encourage you to make notes in your journal after reading each topic, to document your thoughts about what you have just read. This book and your journal are both tools for use in your journey, so make the most of them.

The guidance in this book comes mainly in the form of discussion. The format is meant to help you become aware of techniques that may help you end your crisis, to bring attention to decisions that you will likely be facing and to ease you into issues that may confront you in day-to-day life. In each of these areas, I have shared the knowledge gained through my own experiences as well as from the experiences of others, creating a road map for you to know what might lie ahead and how curvy the road may get. However, as you will come to realize, your experience with HIV is your own to create. Therefore, I have tried not to dictate what your behavior should be but instead highlighted the benefits and drawbacks that I have become aware of for certain courses of action.

Since my primary goal is to help give you direction in your journey towards peace, each discussion is designed to make you aware of the topic, offer some insight and then leave you to consider your course of action in the matter. You are encouraged to use outside resources to find more information about every topic so that you can make fully informed decisions that work for you.

When you read this book, you will notice under some topics a reference to certain medical studies that have been done. I have purposely not included any detailed information about these studies to avoid having you get distracted or overwhelmed by medical information while you are working your way through the stages in this book. If you are interested in reading some studies and can handle the volume of medical information, then you can easily find this type of information all over the Internet, either on websites or in online newsletters. However, I caution you not to do this kind of reading until you have at least completed the first stage of your journey, *Ending Your Crisis,* contained in Chapter 1. It is important that you begin your healing by controlling the amount of information about HIV that you take in right now.

I realize that some of you might not really understand much about HIV or AIDS. While it is important for you to have some basic understanding for use in making medical decisions, reading too much information about HIV or AIDS at this point might do your mind more harm than good. Let me give you a brief overview of the medical aspects involved, just so you will know what doctors or other people are talking about. Take a deep breath, let it out and then read on.

What is HIV and how is it different from AIDS? You have probably seen them written together a lot, especially as HIV/AIDS. HIV is a virus that attacks the immune system and weakens it over time. Primarily, this weakening occurs as a result of immune cells, known as T-cells, being killed off by the virus. The fewer T-cells your body has, the less of a fight it can mount against illness. A person without HIV normally has between 1000 and 1400 T-cells in each cubic milliliter of blood. A person with HIV could have as few as zero T-cells if the illness is quite progressed. When a person has less than 200 T-cells or experiences an opportunistic infection such as pneumonia, an official diagnosis of AIDS is usually given. Viral load is another phrase that you will likely hear mentioned. Viral load is the number of HIV organisms in a cubic milliliter of blood. It can range from one to millions, depending upon how active the virus is within a person and how quickly it is replicating new copies of itself.

Currently, the main treatment approach is to suppress the virus with drugs. Certain medications, when taken in combination, make it very difficult for the virus to replicate. Those people who respond to treatment with drugs generally see their viral loads drop, sometimes so low that the virus is considered undetectable. However, the virus does remain in the tissues of the body and will begin replicating again if not suppressed by the drugs. You can still infect others with the virus during this period. With the decreased viral load, however, T-cells are under less attack and the number of them usually increases. This virus suppression using medications could go on for years, but only if the virus doesn't mutate and adapt to the drugs involved, causing resistance. The drugs themselves can have serious side effects in some people.

This medical version of HIV and what causes AIDS is the most generally accepted one, but you should know that there are other opinions out there. You should also understand that treating HIV with drugs is only one approach among many. There are alternative treatment methods such as natural ones involving herbs and holistic therapy, and complementary treatment methods that use both medications and natural treatments. We will get much further into this discussion when you are ready for it, but for now, I hope that you have a simple understanding of how the virus works in your body. A great resource for understanding HIV medical terminology is the *National AIDS Manual Glossary,* which defines words and phrases associated with HIV and its treatment. Definitions are usually only one sentence long and are written in simple language. Pronunciation guides are even included. Check the resource listings in Chapters 2 or 5 for more information about how to find this free publication. Using this glossary may help you not feel totally lost when you are trying to make sense of HIV medical information.

Now that you are up to speed, let's begin. Your journey towards living in peace with HIV starts now.

Stage 1: Ending Your Crisis

Chapter 1

The Crisis Mind and How to Deal With It

You have recently found out that you have HIV. Maybe it was your family doctor who told you, or a counselor at a confidential testing site. Or perhaps as in my case, you heard it from a telephone counselor after you used an anonymous mail-in home testing kit. Regardless of how gently or harshly the news was delivered to you, most likely you are in crisis. What do I mean by crisis? Well, your mind is probably racing, telling you things like your life is over, you will be dead by Christmas, and that you are going to turn into some kind of freak that no one will love and that everyone will be frightened of. Hopefully not, but that's what my mind told me.

I immediately started projecting my own death—a horrible, ugly, lonely fate that could start at any moment. I eventually worked myself up to the point where I was thinking of ending my own life instead of waiting for that unavoidable and agonizingly slow death I was visualizing. I thought that I might be doing my loved ones and myself a favor. It was a frightening time. Suddenly, the notion of doing anything long term seemed ridiculous. Why should I keep putting money in my retirement plan when I would never live to get it out? A five-year car loan would definitely outlive me. No need to take a new job because I would never last long enough to see it through. A one-year lease on my apartment? Too long. Soon I turned to anger. I was angry that I was going to die, angry at all those people around me that were going to keep on living normal healthy lives while I was dying of AIDS, angry at myself for letting it happen and also at whomever gave it to me. I was also full of conflict, certain on one hand that I was dying, yet feeling healthy and alive and not knowing what to make of it. All those healthy habits that I had adopted—eating right, working out, getting enough sleep, avoiding vices such as drinking, drugs and smoking—seemed to have betrayed me, appearing now to be complete wastes of time. I felt like going out and living fast and dangerously, taking risks with my life just for fun. I was going to die soon anyway, so why not go out with a bang? I had no idea what to do next and no concept of what I should be doing for myself to survive in the short or long term. All I could think about was the stories I had heard about AIDS, those gruesome media images and all the other bad stuff out there that I immediately applied to my own hopeless situation. Does any of this sound familiar to you? If so, you are in crisis, my friend.

Well, the fact that you are reading this book at this moment is a pretty good indication that you are very much alive, just as my writing it proves to me that I am still here five years later. Your life is not over, even though it may feel that way right now. Its value has not diminished. Its meaning has not been lost. You are the same person that you were before you got your diagnosis. Same hopes, same dreams, same soul. Sure, finding out that you are HIV-positive is probably the most shocking thing that has ever happened or maybe will ever happen to you. But we human beings are resilient, adaptive creatures—it is our nature. Yes, your life is going to change, but everybody's life goes through changes over its span. We all do our best to adjust and continue enjoying life. I am telling you, right now, without a doubt, that you have the strength in you to make this adjustment and live in peace with HIV. Believe it.

Once you make it through this crisis period, you will do what so many have done before you—adjust and move on with your life, enjoying each day as we all strive to do. Strange as it may sound, you may discover eventually that this experience has made your life better in some ways. As you work to heal your mind, body, and spirit, you may let go of some things from the past that you are still carrying around with you. So before you make any rash decisions about spending your retirement savings, taking risks with your life, or ending it all, let me share some advice to help you make it through the crisis that now confronts you.

You are about to begin the first of four stages on your way to peace, *Ending Your Crisis*. There is no set time for completing this stage of your journey. It will likely take you weeks or months to do so, maybe even years in a few cases. How long it takes for you doesn't matter. What does matter is that you master every topic in this chapter and move out of crisis. Mastering means not only reading and learning about a topic, but also taking what you learn here and putting it into full practice in your life. That is the only way that you can be fully prepared for the next stage as you continue towards the peace that you seek and deserve.

Before you begin, you have one last thing to do—start a journal. It doesn't need to be anything fancy. A simple notebook will do. You just need a private space where you can capture your thoughts during this journey. You never know which of these feelings and fears may end up being the key that unlocks that healing that you are searching for. Keep this journal in a safe place and, for privacy's sake, don't name it. Now you are ready to begin.

First Thing—Stop and Breathe

It is doubtful that you have had a moment's mental peace since you got your diagnosis. Take one now. Stop, close your eyes and take a deep breath in and out through your nose. Now do it again. I know, you probably feel silly doing this. But focusing on your breathing for just a moment will allow your mind to clear. Remember how good this feels because it is going to be your best defense over the coming days, months, and years as you process what has occurred. In moments of stress, panic, fear, or anxiety, stop and take a breath or two until you begin to function rationally again. It doesn't matter where you are, what you are doing, or whom you are with. Just stop and do it, and don't worry what anyone around you thinks. You can give your mind and body a break with a few simple breaths. You will be amazed at how much this will help you at any given moment.

It wasn't until after I got my diagnosis that I had the first anxiety attack of my life. It came as a complete shock to me, having always viewed myself as the strong, independent survivor-type. The day after my diagnosis, I was reading a magazine for people with HIV while sitting in the waiting room of a therapist that specializes in HIV counseling. After reading a few drug ads that listed potential drug side effects and skimming some horrifying letters from readers about the effects of AIDS, I found myself hyperventilating and sick to my stomach. In my panic, I turned completely white and collapsed onto the floor. I lay there alone, helpless, and gasping for air. I felt weak, humiliated, and defeated, wishing I would just die. When the therapist walked into the waiting room, I jumped up in embarrassment, stumbled into his office, and collapsed into a chair. He sat down at his desk and immediately gave me the best advice of my life: "Stop and breathe." Those three simple words soon became my salvation every time I waited for lab results, whenever I read or saw a story about AIDS, or during those moments when I thought my head was going to explode from the stress of thinking too much. Give yourself a break. Give your mind and body a break. Stop and breathe whenever your mind chatter is working you up into a frenzy. Stop and breathe whenever you feel overwhelmed, when you start projecting what horrors the future may hold, or when your body tells you that it has reached its stress limit. You will be instantly glad that you did. It's free, it's simple, and the benefits to your mental and physical health are priceless. It just might save your life.

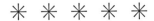

Be Present Focused

Right now, your imagination is your own worst enemy. Most likely, it is projecting a future for you that is full of rejection and vivid horrors. It may be trying to convince you that these terrifying images are true pictures of your agonizing death in the near future. Usually, creativity is something that we desire and embrace in life, but under this circumstance, it could be your undoing. But it doesn't have to be. The truth of the matter is, just as it was before you heard your diagnosis, you don't know what the future holds. None of us does. That fact hasn't changed. What has changed is that your imagination now has some pretty powerful fuel with which to manipulate and amplify all your fears. As a result, it's having a field day. But you have the power to stop it dead in its tracks. All you need to do is to be present focused.

Conceptually, being focused on the present should be easy for us; but in practice, we find it difficult to do. Our minds tend to hang on to the past, digging it up whenever we want to feel happy or sad. On the other hand, we like to get lost in thoughts of the future, daydreaming of what could be someday or what might make us happy later on. But the reality is that the present is the only time that we have, the only time that we have ever had. Nobody can change the past, nor can they control the future. The only time that you can do anything about or have any effect on is right now, the present. That is where your mind needs to be, especially when you are in crisis. It is what you do in the present that helps shape your future. At this point, don't look back and worry about how this happened. You can explore that later, if necessary, when you have your feet more firmly under you. Don't look forward and terrify yourself with wild images of how your life might turn out. Be right here, today, living your life and enjoying what is in front of you at this moment. It is a frame of mind that every one of us could benefit from in life, but so few people ever achieve. Be one of those people, for your own sake.

For right now, whenever you find your mind drifting to the past or the future, stop and breathe to bring your focus back to the present. Focusing on your breathing for just a moment will bring you into the present and clear your mind of the thoughts that plague you. I guarantee that it will make a difference in helping you through this or any crisis.

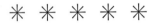

Forgive Yourself

I suspect that in your mind right now, there is plenty of blame to go around. Blame for yourself for letting this happen to you. Blame for whoever might have given HIV to you. Blame for those people who supplied the alcohol or drugs that might have impaired your judgment and caused you to take the risk that led to your being infected. Blame for the condom manufacturer whose product may have failed to protect you. Heck, maybe you even blame for the scientific community for not having already found a cure for HIV/AIDS. Regardless of whom or what it is, someone or something is responsible in your mind for this happening to you. Blame usually leads to anger, and it is likely that anger is also plentiful within you at this moment. Anger is something that you should definitely be concerned about. While blame might cause you some stress, anger is the more dangerous emotion for you to harbor as it can easily turn into hate and violence, either turned inward towards yourself or outward towards those that you blame. It can lead you down a self-destructive path mentally, physically, and emotionally. It may cause you to try and harm yourself through drugs or alcohol or to take unusual risks with your life, including having unprotected unsafe sex. Or it may motivate you to seek revenge against those that you blame, setting yourself up for even more trouble. No good can come from acting out of anger or hate in any shape or form.

The solution to anger is straightforward. Forgive yourself. I know that this may sound too simple to work but it will, trust me. Whatever event that led to your diagnosis happened in the past, and there is no way to ever go back and change it. No matter how much you hurt yourself or others now, the past will never change. Think about that for a moment. Accept it. It's a fact. Blaming yourself in the present only causes you continuing pain and anguish along with the ever-dangerous anger or hate. Accept the blame, forgive yourself and begin living in the present. It truly is the only way for you to make it through this crisis period without causing yourself considerable harm in some fashion.

I know that it is possible that instead of yourself, you only blame others for your infection, therefore making this whole exercise pointless in your mind. Before you skip over this part and move on, let me ask you this—were you involved in the activity or behavior that likely lead to your infection, even in some small way? Did you consent to the sexual contact or choose freely to share a needle with someone? Be completely honest with yourself in answering. It doesn't matter whether or not you knew that the other person had HIV. If you believe, even to the smallest degree, that you chose to be involved in the activity that lead to your infection, then chances are that, somewhere deep inside, you blame yourself for this happening to you. If you don't acknowledge this blame for yourself and bring it out, it will grow and fester over time, turning into that anger and hate that I warned you about. Every time you take your medications, every time you hear the words HIV or AIDS, and every time you have to change anything in your life because of HIV, you will become angry, depressed or, eventually, hateful. That is no way to live. I've seen people stuck in this pattern for years, and it is a miserable existence for them. Take the time now to heal this part of your life by taking the blame, forgiving yourself, and moving forward on your path towards peace.

So now that you've addressed the blame for yourself, what about others that you might blame? How do you deal with that anger? Once you accept your own blame and forgive yourself, you are in a much better position to start forgiving others for the blame that you place on them. You will find that as your anger towards yourself diminishes, so will your anger toward others. I have included a few exercises at the end of this chapter that may help you to start this process of moving past this feeling. This anger is something that you can work out over time, once your crisis has ended and you are more at peace with your situation. For now, focus on yourself. Forgive yourself and allow your healing to start. The rest can wait.

If you find that you can't forgive yourself on your own or that your anger towards yourself or others is too great for you to deal with, I would encourage you to seek some counseling immediately. As I mentioned, I was fortunate enough to see a HIV therapist the day after my diagnosis. Me, asking someone for help—that was a first in my life. But he really showed me how to cut off my anger and self-loathing before it had the chance to blossom into hate, violence, and self-destructive behavior. I did this by forgiving myself. That is not to say that I didn't still have moments of anger after he counseled me. Anger continued to pop up unexpectedly from time to time, causing me stress and anguish. It took me a few years to complete the healing process in that regard. But by getting me to forgive myself early on, he helped me diminish the anger in my crisis mode. Having less anger gave me the chance to continue the long-term healing process on my own without the hate and violence that could have been. Don't spiral down into self-destructive hate and violence. Find the help that you need and deserve to make it through this crisis. You will be glad that you did.

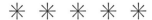

Forget the Stories and Make It Your Own Experience

Oh, the stories. Most of us have seen many tear-jerking stories on television about people living with or dying from AIDS. The media love to play up the melodrama and work our emotions in their quest for high ratings. They parade out the weeping family and friends, crank up the sad music, and show us some horrifying images of people near death. Little do they realize the damage they're causing in those of us who will someday face the same diagnosis. If you didn't see them on television, then maybe you've read them in the paper or heard them from friends. Or maybe you have had the traumatic experience of watching people in your life struggle with HIV or lose their lives to AIDS. These are all powerful images. And right now, your mind is milking each and every one of them to feed your fears and keep you in a panicked state of crisis. Instantly, their stories are your story, your future, your certain destiny. Wow, how does a person overcome that?

The solution again is a simple one. Forget all those stories and make HIV your own experience. It is no different than the rest of life. Did everyone born on the same day as you go on to have the exact same experience in life? Did every person with your physical characteristics go into the same career, live in the same place, or buy the same car that you did? Have they had the same illnesses over time as you have? Of course not. Everyone's life is his or her own experience with its own set of events and outcomes. Yours is no different, even in regards to HIV. What will happen in your future is unique to you, and to a large extent, shaped by how you act in the present every day. Whether or not you believe in fate or destiny, you cannot today determine what the future will hold for you. Don't put your energy into projecting a future that you really know nothing about with any certainty. Instead, put it into living here in the present, enjoying your life at this moment. Pretty soon you will realize that these moments in the present start to string together into what we call our lives, unfolding slowly over time. Believe it. I am living proof. Five years after my diagnosis, my life continues and has evolved in fantastic ways that I could never have imagined when I was in crisis. Had I given up back then, I would have missed out on so many amazing experiences over these past five years as well as the ones that I am certain are yet to come. Don't give up on yourself because of what has happened to others. Remember that your life is your own experience. Live it day by day, in the present. It will make a big difference in your effort to heal.

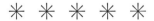

Use Your Support Network

What is a support network? I had to ask myself that same question back when I got my diagnosis. Conceptually, I had always thought it was people in your life who would be on your side when you needed them, helping you without judgment, lectures, or hesitation. Turns out I was right. Problem was that I had never tested mine to find out if it even existed, so I was scared that it wouldn't help me. Turns out I was wrong. Support networks just lie there quietly until that precise moment when you sound the alarm, and then they respond with the help that you need.

Do you have a support network in your life? I bet you do, even if you don't realize it. It takes different forms for each person. For some people, it consists of family members, for others maybe close friends or a mixture of both groups. It might also include a religious counselor, such as a priest, minister, or rabbi. Regardless of its composition, just think of the people that you are closest to in your life and consider telling them one by one. Yes, breaking the news that you have HIV to someone that cares intensely for you can be quite an emotional experience, but the payback to you in your effort to end your crisis is beyond measure and completely worth the emotional impact. I encourage you, however, to limit the number of people that you tell at this point to just those whom you feel will give you the emotional and mental support that you need. You are still in a state of crisis, and dealing with multiple reactions to your news may be overwhelming. Once you get more grounded, there will be plenty of time to tell the other people in your life. For now, just zero in on the ones who will give back in a way that will make a difference in helping you through this turbulent period.

If you still don't feel as though you have a support network, don't feel comfortable using the one that you have, or would like additional support, consider getting a therapist or counselor if you don't already have one. They are impartial, emotionally detached, and experts at listening. Often, they can skillfully reflect back your words in a way that helps you to have self-realizations about the causes of, and solutions to, your current issues. At any rate, just hearing yourself speak about your feelings might be enough for you to recognize what changes you might make to improve your situation. As I mentioned before, the therapist I used helped me immensely. Even though I had a strong support network, additional input from someone who was outside my daily life definitely helped me to gain perspective on what was happening to me and what I needed to do to be okay. You can always give it a try, and then stop if it isn't working for you.

If you live in a country that has national health care, then you should have no problem getting in with a therapist. If you live in the U.S., any insurance plan you might have should cover therapy to some degree. You might also have therapy coverage through an employee assistance plan, if your employer has one. These plans are designed primarily to provide services to employees in crisis. I used this type of plan during my crisis to find a therapist and have my visits covered. Most of these plans are managed by outside contractors who don't usually tell your employer the specific reason why you sought the counseling, so don't be too worried about privacy in this instance. If you don't have insurance, your local HIV/AIDS service organization may be able to provide counseling or make a referral to a therapist that will see you at a reduced rate or on a sliding scale payment basis. The resources are there, so just go and get what help that you need during this time.

There is one more thing for you to consider—use caution in attending organized support groups at this point. From my own personal experience, some of these support group sessions end up being recitals of one horror story about HIV/AIDS after another. I have seen newly diagnosed people turn white and run from the room during such groups, never to return. I don't mean to belittle anyone's experience with HIV or the value of these groups to some people, and not every support group ends up being this way. However, still being in crisis about your diagnosis, you are probably not in the frame of mind to hear other people's troubling tales without using them to project a horrible future for yourself. My advice is to consider skipping these sessions for now, unless you can find a group that is intended only for newly diagnosed people such as yourself. Being among other newly diagnosed people would at least provide the possibility of sharing common fears, feelings, and thoughts with others likely to be in crisis as you are. You may be able to find some comfort, support and healing in the process. Another caution—as wonderful as the Internet is for finding useful information, I would also recommend skipping chat rooms or message boards devoted to HIV/AIDS for the same reasons as above. Once you are out of crisis, your mind will be better equipped to deal with any unsettling stories that you might hear while participating in group support activities going forward.

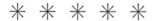

Consult a Physician

If you are anything like I was, you probably feel that you have to see a doctor right this second because every day that you go untreated is another day where you could develop some terrible illness. I had to wait until three weeks after my diagnosis to see a doctor. Three weeks! I don't think I slept more than five minutes in those three weeks, tossing and turning as I thought about all the horrible things that I imagined were happening inside my body. I was certain that I would die at any moment from just about any illness or disease imaginable. Every pain, every cough, every blemish was the onset of something serious waiting to do me in. Can you relate? I'm guessing that you can.

Well, I am here to tell you, HIV doesn't work like that. Unless you were one of those unfortunate few that discovered their HIV infection because of a serious illness such as pneumonia, you are probably in pretty good health. The timeline on HIV is generally one of years, not days, so waiting a few weeks to see your doctor shouldn't kill you. But then again, don't let that be a reason to delay seeking medical advice and treatment. Early intervention with HIV, as with any illness, is often one of the keys to long-term survival. I am just saying to relax if you experience slight delays in getting treatment. Of course, if you really do develop some sort of serious condition, seek immediate medical attention.

You may be feeling afraid or embarrassed to use your regular doctor. Maybe he or she has been your doctor for your whole life, and you don't want to disappoint them with your "mistake." Or maybe you live in a small town and are afraid that your doctor will tell others about your condition. Possibly he or she is your family's doctor, and you are concerned that your family will somehow find out about your HIV. While doctor-patient confidentiality should stop this from happening, in the real world, it is still possible. As I will discuss in Chapter 2, some states in the U.S. allow your doctor to tell your partner or children about your HIV. In the end, you will have to make the decision about which doctor to see based upon on your comfort level with these risks. However, if you decide not to see your regular doctor, find another doctor and go see them. The relief that you will feel from having the attention of a trained professional is invaluable.

For most people, though, the biggest decision is usually whether to see a general physician or a specialist. That is a decision I had to make during my crisis. Though I trusted my regular doctor's medical knowledge, I wanted to have someone looking after me that was devoted full-time to HIV care. I just knew myself well enough to know what would bring me peace of mind. Since you are in crisis right now, don't stress too much about this type of decision. Once you are more grounded, you can take a more active role in managing your health care and medical treatment. For now, if you feel comfortable with your regular doctor, then that's whom you should see. If you already know that you want a specialist, find one that takes your insurance and make an appointment. If you feel comfortable, you might ask any HIV-positive people that you know if they could recommend a specialist to you. If you live in the U.S., you may need a referral from your regular doctor to see a specialist if you have an HMO or other type of managed care plan.

Seeing a doctor should be a no-brainer for most people with HIV, but I know of people who were too afraid or embarrassed to go to any physician and admit that they were HIV-positive. Frankly, you still have HIV whether or not you seek medical attention. Allowing your ego and your pride to stop you from having every chance to live a long, peaceful life with HIV seems like a certain invitation for stress, anguish, and ultimately, regret. Physicians go into practice because of their desire to help and heal people, not to judge or belittle them. Trust them to treat you with respect and caring. Go get the medical attention you deserve and that could really help you during this troubled time.

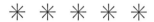

Go on Information Flow Control

People commonly have one of two extreme reactions after they get their diagnosis. Either they completely avoid any mention of HIV, or they seek out, read, and absorb everything that they can get their hands on about the subject. Neither behavior will serve you very well in your present state of mind. You don't want to live in denial about HIV as you have to confront this crisis and work through it, but neither do you want to send your fear-loving mind into information overload with lots of new material to scare the daylights out of you. I suggest that you aim for some middle ground by going on information flow control. Information flow control means that you determine just how much information about HIV is enough for you to digest at any one time. As with most things in life, moderation is the key. Too little and you get nowhere, too much and you could fall apart. Family, friends and doctors might be throwing information at you in an effort to help. It is up to you to set your own limits on what you can handle.

To tackle this challenge during my crisis, I subscribed to a newsletter from Project Inform that keeps tabs on HIV-related medical news and treatments. It seemed like a good idea at the time as the newsletter came out every six weeks, giving me plenty of time to digest its contents without getting overloaded. When my first issue arrived, I let it sit on my desk unopened for two weeks. Then one day I just ran over to the desk, ripped the envelope open and started reading. Within seconds, my heart was racing, I became light-headed and my legs buckled under me, sending me crashing to the floor.

Obviously, the stories about drug side effects and HIV-related illnesses were more than my mind could handle at that point. I started stockpiling the newsletters until a time when I felt that I was in a better place mentally, which came about three months later. Even then, I read them at lightning speed, as though I were trying to get the necessary evil over with as quickly as possible. Yes, my heart still raced a bit, and I did skip a few articles based on their scary titles alone. But this time, I was smart enough to read sitting down! The point of my story is that you are responsible for determining how much information you can handle right now. There is no need to run out and learn everything at once. You will have time to learn more when you are more at peace with HIV. At least for now, just keep your toe in the water to make sure that you don't go into denial about your diagnosis.

Sometimes the HIV information overload can come in the form of a person. Right after my diagnosis, I thought it would be good to make friends with some other people living with HIV. The first person I met had been living with HIV for 13 years and had fully integrated it into his life, an approach I now know is a wise tactic for long-term health and peace. His way of doing this, however, was to relate everything in his life to HIV. Every thought, every action, and every sentence out of his mouth referred to HIV. Even a comment about the nice weather involved HIV. It made me extremely uncomfortable. I knew I wasn't in denial, but I couldn't spend every waking moment thinking or talking about HIV. For my mental health, I knew I needed to focus on other aspects of my life, too. I told him that I couldn't be his friend because of where I was mentally in dealing with HIV. He was very hurt and didn't really understand what was wrong. Still, I had to do what worked for me. I needed to manage the flow of information about HIV that came into my life and into my mind if I ever wanted to end my crisis. To help yourself out of crisis, give some consideration to doing the same.

✳ ✳ ✳ ✳ ✳

Helpful Exercises

It is time to bring your journal to life. When working through the exercises below and in the remainder of this book, be sure to record all your thoughts, feelings and ideas in your journal for use in your healing. Include chapter numbers and section headings in your journal so that you can easily come back anytime and read the information you have captured. This journal is your personal plan for finding peace with HIV and AIDS. Put it into use on your journey every day.

To kick off your journal, take a moment to write down every thought, image, or feeling that you have had since the moment you got your diagnosis. Include every thought you can remember, no matter how bad it may seem. This is your chance to get it all out.

Now that you have them down in writing, you may be surprised at some of the things that you were thinking. But rather than judge yourself for thinking awful or irrational things, take ownership of these thoughts and feelings you're having. They are yours. They are how you feel right now about having HIV. The insight you have just written here will prove to be a valuable tool on your journey towards peace with HIV. Reread it often as you complete this workbook, just as a reminder of where you started from and how far you have come in your progress towards peace.

Take advantage of the exercises below to work through your current crisis and help put an end to it. Don't forget to use all the resources available to you to support your effort here in this stage. These resources include counselors, therapists, HIV/AIDS service organizations, and publications and websites such as the ones listed as examples in the book. You have many tools at your disposal, so use them freely as you work to take control of your crisis mind.

First Thing—Stop and Breathe

You have already learned the basic breathing exercise in this chapter. There are a few variations of this breathing exercise you might also want to try. For the first one, instead of inhaling with both nostrils, just use one. Press a finger up against the right side of your nose, holding the nostril closed. Breathe in through the left nostril, once again focusing on the sound and the feeling. Hold the breath for a moment, then press your left nostril closed and breathe out through the right one. Keep switching back and forth. You get the idea.

The second variation is called the "Breath of Fire." Contrary to what you may be thinking, it doesn't involve eating jalapeño peppers! Inhale deeply through both nostrils, and then when you exhale, do it through your nose in short choppy breaths as you push out the air. It is kind of like panting through your nose. If you do it right, you should feel the muscles in your abdomen tightening.

There are entire books and classes devoted to breath work as a way to reduce stress and improve your health. Regardless of what method that you choose, remember to stop and breathe anytime your mind won't stop, when the stress of life gets too great, or when you need a moment's peace to regain your energy.

Take a moment here to try all three of your new breathing techniques along with any others you might know of. Write down in your journal your results from trying each one. Did any method help you clear your mind? Which one worked the best? How did you feel when you used each one? What variations of breathing can you think of? What was the first thought that popped back in your mind? Did you use a breathing technique to clear it out again? Write it all down.

Practice often and keep a log of your efforts. Soon it will be second nature to use breathing at any moment when you need a break from this or any crisis.

Be Present Focused

The breathing techniques you just learned are excellent ways to clear your mind and stay present focused. Let me share a few more methods for you to try. One is the bubble method. Whenever you find your mind drifting to uncomfortable thoughts of the past or the future, imagine that you are under-water looking up at your thoughts. Now imagine that you are taking those thoughts of the past or future and putting them in bubbles. Let the bubbles float away out of your head as they drift out to sea. It really works. You can't always stop thoughts of the past or the future from popping into your mind, but you can bubble them away once you realize they are there.

Another method for removing these thoughts is to focus on some keywords instead. By keywords I mean things you want in your life right now. For example, whenever you find those past or future thoughts in your head, clear them out by thinking of a word such as *peace*. Focus on *peace* by visualizing the word in your head and repeating it over and over again in your mind. There will be no room for any other thoughts, and your energy will be spent focusing on something that you want in your life right now, in the present. That seems like a good use of energy to me.

Try each of these methods right now to try to clear your mind and bring your thoughts back to the present. Record the results of your effort in your journal. Did any of these methods work? Which one worked the best? How long was it before a thought of the past or future popped back in? Did you use another method to get rid of it? Which keyword did you choose? What others keywords might you use? Again, write down the results.

Practice makes perfect here, so use these methods several times a day to help your mind stay in the present, the same place that you are. Keep a log of your efforts. Soon your crisis mind won't stand a chance.

Forgive Yourself

Someone or something is to blame for your being infected with HIV. I am sure of it. Take a moment to make a list here of everyone and everything that is responsible for this happening to you. In your journal, make three columns. In the first column, list each person or thing that you blame. Use the second column to list the reasons you blame each person or thing in the first column.

Good work. My guess is that everyone on this list is someone that you are angry with as well. It is natural for blame to turn to anger as you process the magnitude of the events caused by these people. Have you thought about acting out against any of these people? Maybe you have already done something. For each person or thing in the first column, write down in the third column what you have done or said to them, or everything that you would like to do or say to them as an expression of your anger.

Maybe it felt good to get that out, or possibly you found it to be a painful exercise. Either way, expressing your anger here may be enough to stop you from going any further with the things that you wrote. If you think doing something physical could help you to release this anger, I have an activity for you to consider trying. For each person listed above, take a piece of paper, put their name at the top and then copy down everything you wrote about them in second and third columns. When you have finished writing, grab the paper with both hands and start angrily ripping it to shreds. You might want to also try verbalizing all your feelings towards them at the same time. Yell out loud! The point is to get these feelings out of you before they grow and turn into hate. Yes, anger may be a dangerous and uncomfortable emotion for you to be holding right now, but hate can destroy your life. If this tearing exercise seems too aggressive for you, try putting each person's name on a balloon and then popping it. This too might help you to start putting the anger behind you. If you decide to try either one of these exercises, stop now and record in your journal how you felt while you were doing it and how you now feel afterwards.

Ok, so maybe you were able to release some of this anger inside you and begin moving forward towards your peace. However, you won't get very far until you stop feeling anger towards the most important person on this journey—yourself. This is why you need to now stop and forgive yourself.

Even if you didn't include yourself in the list of people above, you are where the anger starts and where it will have to end. Take a moment here to forgive yourself for getting infected with HIV. Writing in your journal, tell yourself what past event needs forgiving, and then give yourself forgiveness here in the present. I know it might sound corny, but it is something you absolutely need to do in order to end your crisis.

Keep reading what you have written over and over until you feel the words inside. Keep reading until you truly have forgiven yourself for the past, until you know in your heart that you can't change the past but can only forgive it and move on in the present. Whenever you feel blame, anger, or hate controlling you, come back to these words and read them again until you feel back under control.

If you can't live with the anger that you feel or sense hate welling up within you, get help immediately. Find a therapist, a religious counselor, a support group, or any other type of constructive outlet for expressing your feelings and working through them. Your success in finding peace with HIV depends upon learning how to forgive yourself first.

Forget the Stories and Make It Your Own Experience

Stop and think for a moment about one of the stories you've read or heard about people living with HIV or dying from AIDS. Take a minute to write down what you remember of this story, including all the details and images about it that come to mind.

With your mind in crisis at the moment, it is likely you have taken this story and others and applied them directly to your own future. What images of your future do you have floating around in your head right now? Be as detailed as you can when describing these images. Try to determine if each image came from a story you remembered or if it is one you perhaps created on your own.

So now you know what you are thinking about your future and you know where you might have gotten that vision. But there is still one question for you to answer. How do you know for certain this is your future? Be honest with yourself about your feelings as you write them. It is very important for your healing that you understand why you want to believe this vision of your future. What has convinced you that it is your certain destiny?

I am guessing that last step was difficult or maybe even impossible for you to complete. That's because you don't know exactly what your future holds, just the same as before your diagnosis. You will have to find out what is in store for you by living one day at a time, same as everyone else. But being present focused and living your life from day to day takes practice and some planning. Take a few minutes here to list ways that you might accomplish this task each day in your life. What will help you to think only of today? What will fill you with hope for the future? What you write now will be your plan of action for making your experience with HIV your own.

Use Your Support Network

Your support network consists of those people who support you no matter what. Who are these people in your life? Make three columns in your journal, and then list their names in the first column. Now use the second column to come up with reasons for each one as to why you think that they belong in your support network.

Now that you have your list, stop for a moment and imagine yourself telling each person the news about your status. What can each of these people give you in return that will help you? It is important to consider this because you might want to limit the people that you tell right now to only those that will help you make it through this difficult time. Use the third column to record this in your journal.

A quick review of your list will show you those who might be the most likely to offer you support. Before you pick up that phone, though, you will need to give some thought as to what you are going to say to them and how you are going to say it. Take a moment here to draft in your journal exactly what you will tell them. Consider also the time and place that you will tell them, and whether you will tell them in person, by phone, or in some written form. Once you have your plan together, put it into action and get the support that you need to make it through this crisis.

Consult a Physician

I am certain that you understand the need to see a physician now that you know that you have HIV. But maybe you are hesitating for some reason. What are your fears about seeing a doctor? In particular, what are your fears about seeing your regular doctor, if any?

By acknowledging your fears, you at least now recognize what has been stopping you. Knowing how important it is for you to get medical treatment sometime soon, how will you get past these fears? Will confidentiality laws put your mind at ease? Would it help to see someone other than your regular doctor? Take a moment now to consider what it would take for you to overcome your fears and receive the medical treatment you deserve. Don't be afraid to include using a counselor or therapist to achieve this if you feel you can't do it on your own. Make your plan of action in your journal right now.

You might also be trying to decide whether or not to switch to a specialist for your care. Are you happy with your regular doctor? If so, then why do you want to use a specialist? What benefits do you see for yourself in doing so? Do you see any drawbacks? Make sure that you capture all your thoughts and concerns in your journal.

So now you know what may be driving you on an emotional level towards using a specialist. Now it is time to factor into your decision the cost involved in making this change. If you live in a country that has national health care, then the cost of using a specialist is probably not an issue for you. That means you already have all the information that you need to formulate your plan for

seeing a doctor. However, if you live in the U.S., the cost of a specialist may still be a factor. Does your insurance cover you seeing
one? Will you have to pay extra out-of-pocket expenses to do so?
Will you need a referral from your primary care doctor? Do some
research with your insurance company to see if there is any extra
cost to you, and use your journal to take notes.

In the end, you will have to weigh your feelings from above
against the costs involved and decide what approach is best for
you. Use your journal to analyze whether or not it makes sense
for you to use a specialist right now. Just be sure that your plan
of action for this topic includes seeing a doctor of some type,
regardless of whether they are a generalist or a specialist.

Go on Information Flow Control

How much information are you hearing or reading each day
about HIV? How much each week? Try and describe the current inflow of information, where it is coming from and how
it makes you feel when you take it in.

Right now your mind is likely to take everything that you
hear and read about HIV and turn it into some horrifying
image of your future. Your best bet is to limit the amount of
information that you absorb to just what you can handle at the
moment without creating anxiety or panic. Do you know
where that limit is for you? If not, how will you find out? Take
a moment to write down your thoughts about where your limit
is or ways that you might discover it.

Finding your limit is one thing, but keeping information that you take in about HIV from exceeding that limit is quite another. What is your plan for controlling the amount of information that you take in? How will you deal with media images and stories? What methods will you use to learn about HIV at a speed that is comfortable for you? Think for a moment about what would work for you, knowing how your mind works. As you use your journal to create your plan of action for this area, remember that you are the guardian of your own mind.

Chapter 1 Checklist

Before you leave Chapter 1, complete the following checklist to ensure that you are mentally prepared to begin building a solid foundation for yourself. You can continue on to the next stage in Chapter 2 without having accomplished everything on this list; however, don't forget to come back and finish off your work on these truly important areas. You will need to complete all the tasks here before moving on to Stage 3 in Chapter 5.

Take a page in your journal, and number it from 1 to 37. Every time you finish a step below, put the date that you completed it in your journal next to the corresponding number. Including the headings in your journal may help you to keep track of which specific areas you still need to work on before you can move forward.

First Steps

1. Acknowledged the thoughts, images and feelings that you have experienced since your diagnosis

Stop and Breathe

2. Practiced the breathing techniques listed in the chapter and logged the results

3. Used a breathing technique to clear your mind in a moment of stress or anxiety
4. Using a breathing technique several times each day to give your mind a break

Be Present Focused

5. Identified when your mind was drifting to the past or future
6. Practiced the techniques for staying present focused listed in chapter and logged the results
7. Used a breathing technique to bring your mind from the past or future back to the present
8. Used the bubble method or keyword method to bring your mind from the past or future back to the present
9. Using the above techniques or methods several times a day to stay present focused

Forgive Yourself

10. Identified whom you blame for your HIV infection
11. Recognized what anger you are holding and how it is affecting your actions
12. Accepted that the past can never be changed and that you can only live in the present
13. Forgave yourself for the past in writing, including getting infected with HIV
14. Noticed that the anger within you, both towards yourself and others, is diminishing
15. Considered beginning counseling or therapy to manage the anger or hate within you, especially if you have acted out upon it

Forget the Stories and Make It Your Own Experience

16. Acknowledged the stories that you have heard or read about HIV/AIDS
17. Acknowledged the fears and images your mind is projecting for your future

18. Accepted that you don't know what the future holds anymore than you did before you had HIV
19. Realized that those HIV and AIDS stories you have heard or read are not your story
20. Accepted that your experience with HIV is yours to create each day in the present

Use Your Support Network

21. Identified the people in your support network and why they belong there
22. Identified what you will get in return from telling each person on your list about your HIV
23. Decided what you will say about your status and how you will say it to each person
24. Accepted that you will have to let each person have his or her own reaction to the news, then deal with it
25. Told each person in your support network your news about having HIV
26. Began counseling or therapy if you felt that you needed additional support, especially if you are experiencing depression or anxiety

Consult a Physician

27. Acknowledged your feelings and fears about seeing your doctor
28. Found a way to overcome your fears and seek out medical attention
29. Decided to use your own doctor or located another doctor that your insurance covers and made an appointment
30. Analyzed whether or not you want to see a specialist right now and why
31. Checked your insurance to ensure that specialist visits are covered
32. Saw a doctor about your HIV at least once to get the professional medical attention that you deserve

Go on Information Flow Control

33. Determined how much information you are hearing or reading about HIV on a daily or weekly basis
34. Determined whether you are receiving too much information about HIV and going into information overload
35. Recognized if you are receiving too little information about HIV and slipping into denial
36. Acknowledged that you are the guardian of your own mind and in charge of managing how much information it takes in during your crisis state
37. Managed the inflow of information about HIV by trial and error until you arrived at a flow that is comfortable for you

Resource Examples

Note: As a reminder, this list of books available and other similar lists throughout this book are just a sampling of publications that exist. There are many more resources that you could find by doing a search on your own. My inclusion of a book on any of these lists does not mean I am endorsing or promoting it in any way, or that I have read or used the book on my own journey. Again, the purpose here is strictly informational.

The Transformative Power of Crisis, Robert Alter

How to Forgive Yourself and Others, Eamon Tobin

The Power of Now, Eckhart Tolle

Relating to the Relatives: Breaking Bad News, Communication, and Support, Thurstan B. Brewin

Surviving: Coping with a Crisis, Dr. Bob Montgomery, et al

Forgiveness: How to Make Peace with Your Past, Sidney and Suzanne Simon

Before You Think Another Thought, Bruce I. Doyle

When Your Doctor Has Bad News: Simple Steps to Strength, Healing & Hope, Dr. Al B. Weir and Joni Eareckson Tada

Thoughts & Feelings: Taking Control of Your Moods and Your Life, Martha Davis, Ph.D.

Forgive and Forget: Healing the Hurts We Don't Deserve, Lewis B. Smedes

Fighting for Your Life: How to Survive a Life-Threatening Illness, Jerome Wolfe

The First Year—HIV: An Essential Guide for the Newly Diagnosed, Brett Grodeck and Daniel S. Berger

Note: To find the resources described for any website in this book, you may have to do a search within the website using keywords from the description I've included. Links to the information you are seeking are not always easy to find just by clicking through the website indicated. Also, similar to the book list above, this list is just a sample of available sites and not an endorsement or promotion of those sites. You should definitely consider doing your own search for sites and make you own evaluation of their value to you.

Project Inform, www.projinf.org
Look for: Guidance tailored for the newly diagnosed regarding setting up medical treatment

The Body Positive, www.thebody.com
Look for: Guidance for the newly diagnosed, including articles on how to deal with anxiety

UK Coalition, www.ukcoalition.org
Look for: Step by step guidance for the newly diagnosed, including how to handle emotional issues

Heart of Richmond (Canada), www.heartofrichmond.com
Look for: Brief guidance for the newly diagnosed, including link to a support group

Babes Network, www.babesnetwork.org
Look for: Tips and newsletter for the newly diagnosed, geared towards women

Stage 2: Building Your Foundation

Chapter 2

Important Early Decisions for You

Hopefully, things are getting a bit easier for you by now. Though you may still be in crisis to some small degree, the coping techniques you mastered in Chapter 1 should be helping you to have more frequent moments of peace and clarity. If you keep remembering to breathe and to be focused in the present, you will soon discover these moments increasing until they begin to string together into entire hours and days. It will happen. However, if you still feel deeply in crisis, find yourself filled with anger, or are still unable to control your mind or emotions, stop here and go back to the *Ending Your Crisis* stage in Chapter 1. Ninety-five percent of living in peace with HIV is mental, so take the time now to put a solid mental foundation in place to support this goal. You will only be doing yourself more harm than good by jumping ahead at this point. Besides, there is no timeline for completing these stages, as you have to go at your own pace. Go back and ensure your success in being prepared for the next stage of your journey.

If you feel comfortable with your progress during the first stage in Chapter 1, then you are ready now to begin *Building Your Foundation* over the next three chapters. As you start to get your feet back under you, there are some important decisions that need your attention at this point on your road to living peacefully with HIV. Each of these decisions could be put off until another time if that's what you decide is best for you. But taking the time and energy now to at least consider these important issues will go a long way toward shaping that peaceful future that you are hoping for.

Don't forget to keep using your journal to capture any thoughts that you have or questions you may want to ask someone. Any one of these thoughts or questions may turn out later to be the key to achieving your peace.

Whether or Not to Tell Your Family

The question of whether or not to tell your family members right now may be a very difficult one for you, depending upon how close you are to them, the dynamics involved, and possibly some cultural aspects. By family, I am referring mainly to your parents, brothers, sisters, grandparents, aunts, and uncles. What may be helpful for you to remember is that there is no right or wrong answer here. The only thing you need to consider is what feels right for you today. Tell those your heart calls for you to tell, and save the rest for another time when you are better able to deal with their reactions to your news.

As fate would have it, I had a trip home to Ohio planned for two days after my diagnosis. Though we have never been a close family, I knew it was going to be difficult for me to hold it all in and not tell at least some of them my news, especially my mom. Politically, she's the one in my family I would have to tell first or else face her anger later when she found out that other family members knew before she did. You get the picture. Instead of canceling my trip, I decided to go in hopes of somehow finding support and healing in the process. I don't know what possessed me. I could not comprehend a more horrible fate than having to tell my mother to her face that her baby boy had HIV and might become horribly ill and die at any moment. It was a mother's worst nightmare and the moment I had feared ever since HIV/AIDS was first linked to the gay community. Suddenly, it was my reality.

There I was in her kitchen, telling her the shocking news. Immediately she began to cry. In the middle of her grief, she turned to me and said angrily, "How could you let this happen? I thought you were being safe." Ouch! That cut me straight to the bone. If the therapist hadn't helped me to begin forgiving myself for whatever happened in the past, I am not sure what I would have done to myself after that. As it was, I cried along with my mom, telling her that I'd done the best I could and that all I could do now was deal with the present. The scene went on for a few more minutes and ended with us going our separate ways to deal with what had happened. The next day, to my surprise, my mom was back to her normal, cheery self. Wondering if she was in denial, I asked her how she was doing with the news. She told me she'd been upset at first, of course; but since I sounded so positive and had a lot of hope for the future, she had a lot of hope for it, too. Amazing. Given the chance, people will sometimes blow you away with the amount of their understanding and compassion.

I can't guarantee that your experience in telling family members will turn out as well as mine did. But I can assure you that if you feel it is right for you to tell someone the news and then you do, you will likely feel a sense of freedom afterwards, regardless of what their reaction is. It is like the big secret is out of the bag, and you no longer have to lug it around with you in the relationship. I guess you could say that telling family members is really more about you than about them. You are creating the framework for living in peace with HIV by clearing out the hurdles within your family dynamics. More than likely, these same family members will become a part of the foundation that eventually helps you to live in peace with HIV on a daily basis.

There are few more things to mention on this topic. First, you may have the strong fear that your family will reject you once they hear the news. Your mind may be using this fear to convince you that you will get sick and die alone. Yes, it is possible one or more of your family members may appear to reject you, but this might be their way of getting some breathing room to go off and process the news you've just told them. It is also possible that some family members may never be able to deal with your news and may avoid contact with you indefinitely. The bottom line is that if this type of reaction might be too much for you to handle in your current mental state, then consider not telling your family members at this point. You can always tell them later when you are feeling more grounded and ready for whatever their reaction might be. In the end, you have to make it about you, not them. You are the one who has to be okay with your HIV in the short and long term. Take care of yourself first right now so you'll be ready and able to help them later.

It is possible that in telling your family members about your status, you will also have to disclose other potentially upsetting news about how you might have been infected. Sharing with family facts such as you are gay, have used drugs, or had an affair could lead to a very emotional and stressful experience on its own. Adding news about your HIV infection on top of this might be downright unbearable for you and for them. Give some serious thought as to how such an experience would play out with each family member whom you might want to tell, and be sure to be realistic in your assessment. Are you ready to take on this type of experience right now, given your current state of mind? Only you know for sure.

Don't be surprised if a family member chooses the same moment you tell them your news to share some shocking news of their own, especially since you have just opened up to them. Maybe they too have had an affair, experimented with drugs, or done something else you'd never have guessed in a million years they would do. Imagine—in addition to their reaction to your news, you now have your own reaction to their news to deal with. And if their news is a secret, you'll have the additional burden of lugging it around with you as well. Would you be able to handle taking on something like this right now? Be sure to add this possibility to the mix when deciding whether or not to tell your family members at this time.

Perhaps you want someone to know but find it too difficult to actually tell them the news face-to-face. Or maybe telling them is okay with you, but you don't want to deal with all their follow-up questions at a stressful time such as this. There are ways that you could share this information without having to experience those uncomfortable feelings right away. For example, a friend of mine gave some of his family members the book *Honor Thy Children* because he felt it would help them to understand and accept what someone diagnosed with HIV might be going through. He found that using the book saved him from having to answer most of the follow-up questions that he dreaded, avoiding a large source of stress for him. Perhaps instead of using a book, writing a letter or email would be more comfortable for you. However, be sure to give consideration to the other person's feelings when choosing the method. A close family member may be hurt if they feel you didn't value them enough to tell them face-to-face. Take all of this into consideration, and then go with whatever works for you.

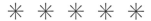

Whether or Not to Tell Your Children

If you have children, it is likely that the first thing you thought of after your diagnosis was how all of this was going to affect them. You are likely trying to decide if you should tell them your news, and if so, how you should tell them. I would guess that you are also thinking about what would happen to them if you became ill or weren't around any more. Rather than try and handle these issues all at once, let's focus now on your decision about whether or not to tell them about your status. Your concerns about who will take care of your children should something happen to you is best discussed later on in Chapter 6, when you have the right foundation under you to consider this kind of topic.

Deciding whether or not to tell your child has to be the toughest choice of the lot. So much goes into such an important decision as this—their age, their demeanor, the dynamics of your relationship with them, their life history, etc. These factors are unique to your life and theirs, and different for every situation and every child involved. I think the best approach for deciding this question is to guess what might happen if you do tell them or if you don't tell them. Using the type of factors above, you may be able to predict fairly well how they may react and how things will turn out if you do tell them. The bigger area of uncertainty here is what will happen if you don't tell them, especially if they find out about your status in a different way. There are several possibilities for you to consider in this area.

First off, kids are curious creatures that tend ask a lot of questions, especially the younger ones. If they see you going to doctor more often or taking new medications, they may figure out that something has changed with your health and become worried. That may result in them constantly asking you about what is happening, a situation that is likely to become a frequent source of stress for you. You might want to also consider that in a few places, your doctor may have the legal right or possibly even the legal obligation to tell your children about your HIV status, especially if your children are also their patients. Finding out this news from someone other than you might be devastating for your children. Also, since you are still dealing emotionally with how to live with HIV, your children are likely to be directly affected by the related changes in your life. They may also be affected by any potential strain in your relationship with a partner, especially if you haven't told your partner about your status. It may be difficult for you to help your children make it through this turbulent time if you haven't told them that your HIV status is the cause of these stresses. Take all these possibilities into consideration and make the best choice that you can for yourself and your children.

If you do decide to tell them about your HIV status, finding the right words might be the most difficult part of the whole experience. Counselors suggest using an approach where you tell them about your condition and that some people do die from it, but that you are taking care of yourself and following the doctor's plan to live as long as possible. Once again, the factors involved are different for every person and their child, so find the words that you think will fit best with your situation. But don't think that you have to go this alone. Contact your local HIV/AIDS service organization for assistance, or ask a doctor, counselor or therapist for some guidance. Use the resources available to make things go as smoothly as possible while dealing with this difficult situation.

Once you do tell your children, it is probably best to keep things at home as normal as possible. To the extent possible, try to continue your normal family routines and rituals to bring an environment of stability to your children's lives. If they seemed troubled, ask your children what they are thinking and discuss their concerns honestly to avoid having them feeling alone. They are going to look to you for the truth and the support they need as they deal with the news. As their parent, you are the best source of both for them during this turbulent time.

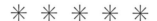

Whether or Not to Tell Your Current Partner

Deciding if you should tell your current partner is definitely an emotionally charged issue. Whether this person is your spouse, your partner, or someone you're dating, there are many factors that you might consider in your decision. First and foremost is the health of the other person. Assuming you have been sexually intimate with this person, they may have been placed at risk of getting HIV. If you continue being intimate with them, then they are definitely being placed at risk, even if you are using protection during sex. Of course, it is possible that this person is the one who infected you, and they may unknowingly have HIV. All these scenarios would seem to be pretty compelling reasons for you to tell them and have them get tested as well.

Perhaps you're thinking of not telling them because you are afraid they will reject you after they find out that you have HIV. Yes, they might do that. But since you are romantically involved with this person, then you are likely concerned about their health and well-being also. I am certain you will balance these concerns and make the right choice for you and for them under these circumstances.

Even beyond the health aspect, your relationship will likely be impacted by your crisis state of mind and the adjustments that you need to make to move towards living in peace with HIV. As you change and adapt, your relationship will need to do the same to keep pace with where you are as a person. If you hide your diagnosis from your partner, you may find yourself becoming increasingly uneasy, frustrated, and withdrawn within the relationship. Your partner may begin to feel these same emotions as he or she senses your withdrawal and discomfort. Also, most newly diagnosed people lose interest in sex for months or even years after being diagnosed. Without knowing the true cause, your partner may take this decline in the sexual aspect of your relationship to mean that things are over between you. Again, go with what feels right for you. But be aware that in some jurisdictions, your physician has the legal right and possibly the legal obligation to tell your partner about your HIV, especially if this person is also a patient of theirs.

Another factor you may want to consider is that it may be a crime where you live to knowingly expose someone to HIV without their knowledge. In other words, once you know you have HIV, you might be breaking the law if you engage in any sexual behavior with someone who doesn't know your status. In this legal circumstance, you can't assume that they either know or can guess your status. You have the obligation of telling them directly to avoid violating many of these laws. I am not certain if this obligation to tell would apply in cases where the other person already had HIV, but you might not want to be the one who tests the court system on this point. Of course, as with any law, while it takes a lot of proof and a burning desire on the other person's part to see you prosecuted and convicted, the possibility does exist. Just the stress of worrying about someone prosecuting you is enough to justify giving strong consideration to telling your partner about your status. You may want to contact your local HIV/AIDS service organization for guidance on what laws exist concerning the disclosure issues mentioned above.

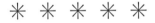

Whether or Not to Tell Your Friends

You may have already told some of your friends about your news as part of your support network. The difference in dynamics with friends as opposed to family may make this easier for you. Your family members are set by birth or marriage whereas your friends are in your life by your own choice. Accordingly, your fear of rejection by your friends may be much less than you felt with your family. Those common elements that brought you together as friends and that connection that you feel with them could make them wise choices for confidants about your status. They are likely good candidates for your support network as well. Everyone's situation is different, so give yours some thought and use it to your best advantage.

When I started telling my close friends, I would try to control their reactions. I would first tell them my news, and then, before they could react, I would say that everything would be okay and tell them not to get upset. This seemed to be an effective method for controlling their reactions, which pleased the "control freak" in me. This approach for sharing my news worked well with the first two people. But when I told a third friend not to be upset, she swiftly cut me off and demanded that I stop telling her how to feel. She sternly reminded me that it wasn't fair to drop a bombshell like this on people and then attempt to stop them from having their own reaction. Yikes! Busted. In an effort to avoid having to experience any unexpected discomfort in telling people, I was stopping them from expressing their own feelings about the news. It never occurred to me that I was disrespecting them by not letting them react honestly.

The lesson for me and for you is to not tell a person unless you are prepared both to let them react and then to deal with their reaction. Otherwise, you aren't being fair to them, or to yourself, for that matter. If you don't show respect for your friends' feelings in this process, you risk losing their friendship and support at a time when you may need them the most. Give this some thought in deciding when to tell people in your life. There is no rush.

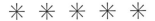

Whether or Not to Tell Past Partners

Logically, it should be easier to tell your news to a past partner rather than your current one because of the lack of a romantic attachment. Of course, how often does life really follow logic? Before you make any decisions about telling these people, let's

figure out who might be on your list to tell. First question—
how far back should you go when making this list? At this point
on your journey, I would recommend limiting the list to persons you have been intimate with between today and six
months before your last negative HIV test result. Six months
is the controversial-yet-generally-accepted time frame for how
long it might take the HIV virus to show up on a blood test
after you have been infected. Once you've identified the proper
period of time, make a list of everyone you can remember
being intimate with during that span. For some of you, there
may be only one person on your paper. For others, it could be
quite a list. Regardless of the number of names involved, if
your intent is to tell those most at risk of having been exposed
to HIV by you, then these are the people we are talking about.
If you've never been tested before, the cutoff point for your
time line becomes much murkier. Just use your best judgment
along with your sense of fairness in deciding whom to include
on this list. Don't use this length of this list of names as a tool
to judge yourself and your behavior in the past. What is done
is done, and you can never change the past. Just focus your attention on the task at hand and do what you need to do for
yourself here in the present.

Once you have your list together, stop for a moment and
consider your mental state. If you think you're not able to handle telling your past partners about your HIV right now, then
don't do it. Wait until another day in the near future when you
feel better equipped to deal with their reactions. You have to
take care of yourself first.

During this process, you may be wondering why you
would want to contact these people at all and tell them anything. More than likely, they are out of your life for a reason,
and contacting them again is not something that you would be
inclined to do. That definitely makes sense. However, let me
suggest a few reasons why you would want to make the effort
anyway. The first is that you may have infected them with HIV
during your intimate behavior with them in the past. Even if
you don't know for sure, you might feel a certain sense of responsibility to at least let them know about the risk so they can

get tested and seek treatment if necessary. Whether or not you parted on good terms, I have no doubt that you are a compassionate person who cares for all people in this world, and this caring would include the people on your list. Let me give you another way to think about it. If the situation were reversed, would you want someone to tell you? I know I would so that I could get treated as early as possible and improve my chances for a long, happy life.

There is another reason you might want to tell these people. It could benefit your health as well. If it turns out that one of these people already had HIV when you were intimate, then they might have been the one who infected you. Knowing what HIV medicines that they were taking at the time could assist you in structuring a more effective treatment program for yourself. Without going into the medical aspects, it might give your HIV a history of sorts to use in more successfully managing your care. Give it some consideration.

So even though you know the people you might want to tell, what if you can't find them? What if they've left town with no forwarding address? What if you only knew their first name or no name at all? What if you were on vacation halfway around the world and knew you'd probably never see that person again? All good questions. The answer here is to make the amount of effort with which you are comfortable in regards to finding the people on your list. If you don't have or can't find any contact information for a person, then you are most likely at a dead end. Don't beat yourself up about it. Instead, consider promising yourself that if you do someday manage to run into that person or hear that they are around, you will make another effort then to tell them. Or if you feel comfortable doing so, contact your local health department or local HIV/AIDS service organization to see if they could assist you in finding these people. Just remember, the most important person for you to take care of right now is yourself. Decide what you are comfortable doing, make an honest effort to do it, and then move on.

Let's say you've found someone on your list. Now what do you say? Actually, I found that it is not exactly *what* you say but *how* you say it that influences how the interaction might go.

The majority of people I contacted became instantly defensive upon my giving them the news. They thought I was accusing them of giving me the HIV. One person even went so far as to say that he had a negative test a few days before we were together, so it couldn't possibly have been him who had infected me. Yeah, so did I, I told him. But four weeks later, I was HIV-positive. Unfortunately, that conversation ended with a nasty exchange of words. To avoid this type of situation, my advice to you is to cushion the blow as much as possible. Consider starting your news with a statement about this not being an accusation but rather you wanting to do the responsible thing because you may have put them at risk. The truth of the matter is that they might have been the one who put you at risk, and this fact might come out in their response to you. But if they don't volunteer this information, you will have to decide whether it is worth the risk of confrontation to ask them this question about their status. Considering your current state of mind, you might want to save your energy by sharing your news and ending it after their response. At that point, your responsibility to them and to yourself will be done.

If you have remained friends with some of your past partners since you stopped dating, then maybe you have already told them as part of your support network. Lucky you! If, however, you ended a relationship on unpleasant terms, then it may be quite an emotional experience to contact that person for any reason, let alone to tell them this kind of news. So what should you do? You probably know what I am going to say. You need to do what feels right for you. Consider all the factors I have mentioned in this section, weigh them against the potential emotional impact of telling this person, and then make your own decision. I am sure it will be the right one for you at this moment.

$$* \quad * \quad * \quad * \quad *$$

Should You Go on Medications or Not

Let me tell you up front that anything I tell you here will probably be the source of some controversy. Still, I believe it's important for you to get a straightforward picture of what you're facing in this area so you can make the right choice for you. As you will see, change is a big part of HIV treatment and medications. Whatever your choice, it will definitely not be the last one you make concerning medications in your treatment.

What you will learn about HIV treatments is that every approach or protocol has as many supporters as opponents. Some people believe that the "cocktail" of HIV medications is the only way to live long term with HIV. Others believe the drugs are more dangerous than the virus, recommending instead the use of more natural treatments along with lifestyle changes and mind healing. Still others think that a combination of medications and natural methods is the best approach. Unfortunately, these widely differing views leave you right in the middle of the controversy, probably drowning in confusion. How can you make the right choice for you with all this conflicting information coming at you? Good question. Let's take a brief look at two different approaches to treatment.

The allopathic medical community, composed of what you think of as regular doctors, is geared towards treating most illnesses or conditions with pharmaceuticals, the fancy word for drugs. The primary weapon used by doctors for treating HIV is a triple combination of medications dubbed the "cocktail." Devised in the mid-1990s, this combination has greatly improved the prognosis of many people who were struggling with AIDS. The allopathic community has established protocols or standards for when someone should start taking HIV medications. As new information emerges, these protocols have shifted to reflect the new research. Critics point out that some people who began taking medications in prior years would never had been started on the drugs if current protocols had been in effect. Given the number of serious and unpleasant side effects that HIV medications cause in some people, taking medications you might have been able to avoid becomes an important and contentious issue. Also, once you start taking these medications, the common allopathic view is that you can never completely stop without serious risk. I will address this stopping option more in Chapter 5, but for now, just know that there is some debate over whether or not this is true.

The holistic or natural medical community generally believes that pharmaceuticals are more harmful than HIV itself. This community's approach to treating HIV is to use the natural healing properties of plants and other organic materials to treat and heal the body, mind, and spirit. This branch of medicine has been in practice for thousands of years in different parts of the world. One of its core beliefs is that using the whole plant or organic compound in treatment brings out more healing properties than using only one element of these compounds, as many pharmaceuticals do. Incorporated in holistic treatments is healing of the mind, which some holistic practitioners believe is the source of all disease within the body. Therefore, holistic approaches don't just treat the symptoms in the body but also focus on eliminating the source of the discomfort that is disrupting the balance between mind, body, and spirit. Critics have charged that holistic methods lack data to support their validity as effective HIV treatment methods and that people may be damaging their long-term survival chances by not using proven pharmaceutical instead.

So where does this leave you in your immediate decision about whether or not to start taking medications? I suggest you begin by having a lively discussion about the subject with your doctor. Ask your doctor about the protocols, how your lab results fit into them, and what the doctor recommends that you do. Be sure to ask about other treatment options including those that don't involve pharmaceuticals. And don't forget to ask about the side effects of any medications he or she recommends that you take. You might feel comfortable accepting your doctor's recommendation; but if not, you may want to get a second opinion from another doctor. Another idea is to consult your local HIV/AIDS service organization to see if they have an opinion about your doctor's suggested treatment option. Also, if you can handle the information inflow, you might want to search the Internet for any articles about the recommended medications and treatment option. After you research the allopathic options, consider exploring more about holistic methods. You can find information by reading books, surfing online or consulting a herbologist or other type of holistic practitioner. Your local HIV/AIDS service organization may be able to help you find this information as well. Remember to use caution when researching treatment approaches so you don't end up reading or absorbing articles that send you into panic or anxiety, something your mind is still likely to do at this point.

To cut to the chase, unless you are in the midst of a serious HIV-related illness or have been diagnosed with AIDS, don't feel pressure to start taking HIV drugs today, no matter what some people may be telling you. In fact, if you have any serious reservations about starting on drugs, take that as a sign that you need more time to process all the information you've read or heard. Some people don't take medications at all unless their lab results show that their immune system has begun to weaken significantly over time. It is your decision to make, and yours alone. Don't rush it. As always, trust your instincts about what is right for you.

If you do decide to start taking medications but find you can't afford them, contact your local HIV/AIDS organization and ask about public programs that provide the HIV drugs for free for lower-income people. I will give you more details about these programs in Chapter 4 when you are better prepared to deal with managing your medical treatment.

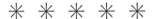

Should You Keep Working or Go on Disability

Back when HIV/AIDS was first emerging and long before the "cocktail" was developed, most people who were diagnosed went onto disability almost immediately. This was due mainly to the limited treatment options and the resulting rapid progression of the disease. In effect, most people were preparing to die. In the mid-1990s, however, the disease's progression in those infected was slowed considerably by use of the "cocktail" treatment approach. As a result, people have started to stay healthy for much longer than before, and more people have continued working after being diagnosed. In essence, people are now preparing to live.

Unless you are suffering from a serious HIV-related illness, you have probably been working since you got your diagnosis. In a way, working might be helping you to adjust during this difficult time. I know that when I was at work after my diagnosis, my mind was occupied with work thoughts as opposed to spending its time torturing me with ugly scenarios of my future. Since my job was low stress, I basically threw myself into my work for a period of time as a defensive measure, working extra hours, taking on additional projects, and keeping my mind as busy as I could. I am not advocating the same path for you, but if you find work to be a healthy distraction for your mind right now, you should probably go with it. Work might also give you a sense of purpose and meaning in your life at a time when your mind might be trying to convince you otherwise.

On the other hand, you might need a break from work if the stress of your job is too much for you to handle right now. If you have sick, personal, or vacation days available, maybe you should take them. If you need more than a few days off, look into your company's short-term disability plan if they have one. Though the terms vary from employer to employer, most short-term disability plans consider HIV in combination with stress to be disabling, which would qualify you for benefits. If your employer doesn't have a plan, you may have coverage from the state or province that you work in, though these benefits are typically less generous. Keep in mind that short-term disability benefits are usually less than your regular pay, probably as an incentive for you to get well and return to work.

In the U.S., it used to be fairly easy to get HIV-related long-term disability benefits from employers or state and federal programs. With the advancements in HIV treatment, however, the outlook for those diagnosed has improved considerably, resulting in much higher hurdles for claiming benefits. Currently, to qualify for benefits, you need to demonstrate how HIV has rendered you unable to work in *any* capacity. Luckily, that is not the case for most of us in relation to our

HIV, as we can go on working and supporting ourselves. But if you feel you have been rendered physically unable to work again, consider filing claims for long-term disability benefits with your employer as well as with state, provincial, and federal programs. Local HIV/AIDS service organizations generally can assist you with filing these claims.

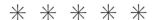

Should You Have Safe Sex or Not

At this point in your journey, sex may either be the furthest thing from your mind or something you find yourself suddenly wanting a lot of. Regardless of which of these two options describes you best at this moment, a discussion about the dating and social aspects of having HIV is best left to a later time, in Chapter 5, when you are more mentally prepared to manage your daily life with HIV in it. That chapter also includes a lengthy discussion about safe sex and its practice. However, if you are being sexually active now, you should consider taking a moment here to analyze your current safe or unsafe sex behavior.

It is common for newly diagnosed people to believe that now that they have HIV, they can safely have unprotected sex with other HIV-positive people or with HIV-negative people that don't seem to care about getting infected. This train of thought seems to come from the idea that once a person has HIV, there is nothing left to protect themselves from. Unfortunately, this notion is far from the truth. Besides the risk of being re-infected with another strain of HIV, you could end up with one of many other sexually transmitted diseases, including hepatitis, syphilis, gonorrhea and herpes. Each one of these that you pile on your immune system takes your health down that much further.

Before you begin making unsafe sex your new practice, talk with a physician, counselor, therapist or a HIV/AIDS organization staff member about the risks of that unsafe sex could present for you. If your goal is to find a way to live a long-term, healthy life now that you have HIV, taking on other diseases or new strains of HIV now may lead to regret down the line. Eventually finding your peace with HIV won't do much to stop the decline in your health these added illnesses will bring on over time. We can talk more about this in Chapter 5, but for now, strongly consider putting off a decision to have unsafe sex until a time when you are able to more clearly understand and accept the serious risks involved.

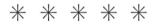

Helpful Exercises

Whether or Not to Tell Your Family

Telling family members that you have HIV may be the thing we all fear the most. What are your feelings and fears about telling your family members you have HIV? Are you afraid of being rejected? Do you have to tell them other news at the same time, like you're gay, had an affair, or used intravenous drugs? When you think of telling them, how do you feel emotionally and physically?

Taking your feelings and fears into consideration, who in your family do you specifically want to tell? Why do you want to tell each person? Make three columns on a page in your journal. Use the first column to list the family members you want to tell. In the second column, write the reasons you want to tell each person listed your news.

Knowing these family members as well as you do, stop and think about how they might react to the news. By the news, I mean all the news you may need to share in order to explain how you got infected with HIV. How do you think each they will react? In the third column in your journal, make your best guess about each person's likely reaction to your news. Be careful not to sugarcoat their reactions in your head, as the goal here is to prepare you for what might really happen.

You are almost there. Now imagine you're prepared to tell each person on your list. How will you do it? What will you say? Will you do it face-to-face, on the phone or in a letter? If your goal is to somehow lessen the impact of your news, then how you say it may be more important than what you actually say. Stop for a moment and use your journal to capture what you might say to each person and how you will say it.

Great! Now you have it all planned out. You know who you want to tell, how they might react, what you will say to them, and how you will say it. Before you being sharing the news, sit down and take a long, hard look at the plan you have just created. Are you ready to deal with each person's reaction? Are you more nervous about some than others? The bottom line here is that if you don't feel that you could deal with someone's reaction in your current state of mind, then don't tell that person right now. It can wait until another time when you are much more grounded and have moved further down your path towards peace. You need to look after yourself right now. Go back to your list and write the word "now" or "later" next to each name to remind you of whom you have decided to tell now or to wait to tell later.

Whether or Not to Tell Your Children

If you don't have children, then skip to the next section. If you do have children, what are your feelings and fears about what will happen to them now that you have HIV? How do you think they will be affected?

There is no easy answer to the question of whether or not you should tell them now. Only you can make that call. However, taking some time now to analyze the pros and cons may help you in arriving at a decision you can live with. As a first step, list the names of each of your children in your journal, leaving plenty of room under each for you to make notes. Now consider things such as their age, their mental state, their personalities, their life history, and your relationship with them. Analyze and record every factor you think might be relevant to your decision on this important matter. Make sure your list for each of your kids is complete before moving forward.

Good, you have the all the facts lined out. Now it's time to bring your imagination into the equation. For each child of yours, imagine how they would take your news. Visualize yourself telling them and them reacting to what you are saying. What do you see? Are their reactions completely different? How do you feel about what you are imagining? Could you tell one child but not the others? Capture everything in your journal.

It is time to turn the tables now. What do you imagine happening if you don't tell your children? More specifically, how will they react if they figure it out on their own but don't hear it from you? Will they be scared and afraid to tell you that they know you're sick? How about if they learn about your HIV by overhearing someone talking to you about it? How will they react to that? How will you react if they are constantly asking you questions about your health?

That is a whole lot to think about, I know. But I'm sure that the welfare of your children is foremost on your mind and worth the mental gymnastics required for you to make an appropriate decision on this important matter. You don't have to go it alone, however. Definitely use the assistance of a counselor, therapist, or doctor if you want some support and guidance in this process. Once you've made your decision, write it in your journal along with the reasons why you made this decision.

If you have decided to tell one or more of your children, how will you do it? What will you say? When will you say it? What will you do afterwards to let them know everything is okay? How will you support their dealing with the news over time? How will you keep your family routines as normal as possible?

Again, get any assistance that will help you to work out your plan. Your children will need your support and love going forward no matter what you decide. Make certain you've made your peace with your choice so you can be there for them now and in the future.

Whether or Not to Tell Your Current Partner

In this context, partner could mean your spouse, long-term lover, or someone you have been seeing for a short time. Basically, it is the person you were involved with when you got your diagnosis. What are your feelings and fears about telling this person that you have HIV? Are you afraid of being rejected or being judged? Do you have to tell them other news as well, such as you had an outside relationship or used intravenous

drugs? When you think of telling them, how do you feel emotionally and physically? Use your journal to explore your feelings and fears about telling them.

This person is important to you if they are still in your life.
Are you concerned that they may have HIV too? That you may
have given HIV to them or possibly they gave it to you? Are
you worried that either possibility will end your relationship if
the truth comes out? If you don't tell them, what effect do you
think that will have on the relationship? Lots of important
questions here for you to answer in your journal.

So now you have a handle on what you are feeling and what
may happen to your relationship if you do or don't tell this person. Now comes the difficult part—deciding whether or not to
tell them. Only you can come up with the right answer here.
Review what you wrote in your journal, look at what is in your
head and your heart right now, and then make your decision.

If you do decide to tell your current partner, what will you
say to him or her? How will you say it? How soon will you discuss this? And what will you do if it appears that you are being
rejected? Take some time to finalize your plan in your journal
to ensure that you keep moving forward on your journey.

Whether or Not to Tell Your Friends

You may have less fear of telling your friends than your family
simply because your friends are in your life by your own choice.
What are your feelings and fears about telling your friends that
you have HIV? Are you afraid of being rejected? Do you have
to tell them other potentially shocking news at the same time?

When you think of telling your friends, how do you feel emotionally and physically?

Considering your feelings and fears, which friends do you specifically want to tell? Why do you want to tell each person? Make three columns in your journal, listing in the first column the friends you want to tell. Next, put in the second column the reasons you want to tell each of them your news.

Knowing these friends as well as you do, think about how they might react to the news. How do you think each person will react? Be honest with yourself to help avoid any uncomfortable surprises. Use the third column to record their potential reactions.

Will you tell your friends the same way you told your family? Will your approach or words used be different? Take a moment to capture what you might say and how you will say it. Include whether you will say it in person, over the phone, or in writing.

Again, your plan is in place. Can you deal with your friends' reactions in your current mental state? Just as you did for your family members, go back to your list and write the word "now" or "later" next to each name to remind you who you've decided to tell now and those you will tell later.

Whether or Not to Tell Your Past Partners

In theory, it should be easier to tell a past partner than your current one because they are just that—in the past. Being in the past, however, doesn't mean there aren't still emotions attached to thoughts of and interactions with that person. What are your feelings and fears about telling past partners that you have HIV? Are you afraid of being judged or accused? Was your breakup with some of them painful or uncomfortable? Be sure to record everything you are thinking and feeling about this right now.

Before you make your decision concerning telling your past partners, you may want to first identify exactly which people we are talking about. Creating a timeline in your journal is a good first step in this process. Your timeline should start today and run back to six months before your last negative HIV test. If you've never been tested before, just pick a date in the past that makes sense to you and seems fair.

Once your timeline is in place, you are ready to make a list of the people to be included. Who were you sexually active with during this time? Are there other people whom you could have exposed through non-sexual behaviors such as sharing a needle while injecting drugs? Give it some deep thought and make the list in your journal. The list may be empty or it may be bursting at the seams with names. You may only know a person's first name or no name at all. In this case, try to put down any kind of identifying information that you can remember, the place that you met, or some characteristic about them. Don't use the length of this list to judge yourself. What is in the past is done, so just focus on the task at hand.

You may continue to think of people over time, so just add to the list as you remember them. Using the names you already have, which of these people can you find easily? Are there those you know you'll never be able to find? Mark those people that you can find easily with the word "found" and the others that you will never find with the word "never." Now your real work begins. Can you find the remaining people on the list? Maybe you can find them using the phone book, through a mutual friend, or back at the place where you first met them. Perhaps you see them online from time to time. If you are comfortable asking for help, it is possible that your local health department or local HIV/AIDS service organization may help you to find these people. Use your journal to make notes during your search. If a person has moved out of town, had their phone number unlisted, or are in some other way unreachable, then don't worry about it. Just make an honest effort to find them, and if you don't, vow to tell them if you happen to cross paths later or if you hear that they are back in town. Label these people as "later" on your list.

So now focusing on the people that you have found, what will you say when you talk to them? Perhaps you would prefer to say nothing at all to them, especially if your breakup was not a pleasant one. You will have to decide for each person whether or not you can handle talking with him or her right now. For those whom you do decide to contact, give some thought as to what you will say, how you will say it, and how you think they will react. Take a moment here to create your plan for making this happen. Having the words written down and ready for use might make this an easier experience.

Should You Go on Medications or Not

This is a difficult question to help you with, I must admit. It is such an important and personal choice. Let me start by asking you this—what have you heard or read about HIV medications? What side effects have you heard of? What feelings and fears do you have about taking HIV medications? What fears do you have about not starting on HIV medications?

At least now you know where you stand emotionally about starting HIV medications. Unless you have a serious HIV-related illness or your immune system is extremely weak, there is probably no need to rush your choice of treatment options. My best advice is to do diligent research on all the options before choosing one. Just be careful not to go into information overload as your mind may be just waiting for juicy information to use in scaring the daylights out of you.

Here is a suggested checklist to follow when researching and investigating treatment options. You may decide to skip some items or add some of your own. Number a page in your journal from 1 to 12, and then record the date you complete each step that you choose to undertake. Be sure to use this journal page to take good notes about treatment options as you do your research. When you're finished, use all the information that you gathered to make your decision about whether or not to start medications now.

1. Discuss your lab results with your doctor and get treatment recommendations.
2. Ask your doctor about treatment options that don't involve medications.
3. Ask your doctor about the potential side effects of recommended medications.
4. Obtain a second opinion if you don't feel comfortable with your doctor's recommendations.
5. Check the Internet for the latest information about the recommended medications and their side effects.
6. Check online for the latest protocols or standards for when to start a person on medications.
7. Contact your local HIV/AIDS service organization for possible guidance about the recommended medications.

8. Ask people already taking the recommended medications about side effects and their overall experience taking them.
9. Research holistic and complementary treatment options on the Internet and through books.
10. Contact holistic practitioners in your area to find out more about what they do and how it can help you.
11. Contact your local HIV/AIDS service organization for guidance on holistic and complementary treatment methods.
12. Ask people already following holistic and complementary treatment methods about their overall experience with these methods.

Should You Keep Working or Go on Disability

If you have been working since you got your diagnosis, how does it feel to be at work right now? Is it more stressful than usual? Is work keeping your mind off having HIV? Are you worried about coworkers somehow finding out about your status? How does your body feel?

If your job is low stress and it helps take your mind off of HIV for part of the day, then maybe you should just go with it. If, however, you have reached your stress limit or feel uncomfortable at work, consider taking some time off. You might just need a few days, or perhaps you need a longer break. Here is a suggested list of benefits to check for and use to get some time off. List each type of time off in your journal, and then write next to it the number of hours or days that you have available to use for that category. If there are any restrictions on using a particular type of leave, be sure to note it in your journal for use in planning any time off.

Personal Days
Sick Days
Vacation Days
Medical Leave (Paid)
Medical Leave (Unpaid)
Leave of Absence (Paid)
Leave of Absence (Unpaid)
Short-term Disability (Employer Plan)
Short-term Disability (State/Provincial Plan)

While doing your planning, keep in mind that disability benefits are usually only 55-65% of your normal pay before taxes. However, most disability benefits are not taxed as income, so compare them to your normal after-tax pay when assessing any financial impact you might experience from using them. Putting aside the financial aspects for a moment, stop and think about the idea of you going on disability. What are your feelings and fears about this? Are you comfortable taking a break to get yourself and your health in order? Or do you feel that you are not truly disabled and are somehow cheating by using these benefits? Are you afraid that labeling yourself disabled will cause your attitude and life to change? Are you worried what others might think? Get it all down in your journal for use in making your decision.

You have all the information you need to make your decision. You know how you feel about working, what your time off options are, and how you would feel about going on disability. Use these three pieces of information to create a plan of action in your journal that fits your life right now. Regardless of what you decide now, remember that you can always change your mind in the future.

Should You Have Safe Sex or Not

Has your interest in sex increased, decreased or stayed the same since your diagnosis? What are your feelings when you think of having sex now that you have HIV? If you have been sexually active, how did you feel during sex? Take a moment here to capture in your journal all your current emotions around having sex.

Hopefully your writing has given you a pretty clear picture of your state of mind when it comes to sex. Now let's turn our attention to your sexual practices. Do you know for sure which sexual practices are safe or unsafe? How do you know? Do you think your idea of safe sex may have changed since your diagnosis? Many people end up confused about what safe sex is after getting infected with HIV through sexual contact. Answer all these questions in your journal now to see where you are in your understanding of safe sex.

Whatever your current idea of safe or unsafe sex for yourself, it might be best to confirm your understanding with a professional in the field, like a physician, counselor or case worker. New studies and information on this topic come out all the time, and staying current on safe versus unsafe sex practices can only benefit you in the long run as sex becomes a part of your life again. Also ask these people what the risks are from having unsafe sex, just so you know what you might be taking on if you have it.

Ok, now is the time to put it all together and understand what safe or unsafe things you are doing or want to do and why. Use your journal now to paint a picture of your current desires regarding this topic and how you think acting on them would affect both your mental and physical health. Once you have done that stop for a moment and think about whether or not you are in the right space mentally to clearly understand and accept the serious risks that unsafe sex could present to you. Is this decision something better made at a later time when you feel much more secure and stable and able to give this serious topic the full consideration it deserves? Finish your work here in your journal by making your decision on what sexual practices you will follow and how doing so will benefit your emotional and physical health in the long run. You can come back and re-evaluate your decision later when you reach Chapter 5.

Chapter 2 Checklist

Before you move on to Chapter 3, complete the following checklist in your journal. It is important that you accomplish each item listed to build your foundation for that lasting peace with HIV that you are seeking. You will need to complete each step below *before* you reach the next stage in Chapter 5. Take a page in your journal, and number it from 1 to 46. Every time you finish a step below, put the date that you completed it in your journal next to the corresponding number. Again, including the headings in your journal may help you to identify which areas still need more of your attention before you can move forward.

Whether or Not to Tell Your Family

1. Acknowledged your feelings and fears about telling your family members about your HIV and how you got it
2. Identified which family members you want to tell, why you want to tell them, and how you think they will react
3. Decided how you will tell them and what you will say
4. Decided whether or not you could handle a reaction that appeared as though you were being rejected

5. Used all the above information to decide which people to tell now or later

6. Told the family members you wanted to tell now

Whether or Not to Tell Your Children

7. Acknowledged your feelings and fears about how your having HIV will affect your children

8. Identified all the factors to consider in deciding whether or not to tell each of your children about your diagnosis

9. Imagined how each child would react if you did tell them and what might happen if they found out from someone else or figured it out on their own

10. Decided whether or not you will tell each child about your HIV

11. Decided how you will tell them and what you will say (if you decided to tell your children)

12. Received support and guidance from a counselor, therapist or doctor, if needed, when making this decision and figuring out how to tell your children

13. Created your plan for keeping things as normal as possible and supporting your children's emotional needs after you tell them

Whether or Not to Tell Your Current Partner

14. Acknowledged your feelings and fears about telling your current partner about your HIV and how you got it

15. Acknowledged the potential effects on your relationship and your children if you do tell your current partner or if you don't tell them

16. Recognized the legal risks of not telling your current partner and the possible right of your doctor to tell them

17. Decided what you will say, how you will say it, and when you will say it

18. Decided how you will handle a reaction that appeared as though you were being rejected

Whether or Not to Tell Your Friends

19. Acknowledged your feelings and fears about telling your friends about your HIV and how you got it
20. Identified which friends you want to tell, why you want to tell them, and how you think they will react
21. Decided how you will tell them and what you will say
22. Decided whether or not you could handle a reaction that appeared as though you were being rejected
23. Used all the above information to decide whom to tell now or later
24. Told the friends you wanted to tell now

Whether or Not to Tell Your Past Partners

25. Acknowledged your feelings and fears about telling your past partners about your HIV
26. Used a timeline to identify past partners to tell
27. Recognized that your mental and emotion health comes first when deciding how many people you can handle telling right now
28. Decided whether or not you are able to handle this process in your current state of mind
29. Made an honest effort to find every person on the list, including seeking outside help (if you feel okay with that)
30. Decided what you will say and how you will say it, including if you will ask about their status at the time you were together
31. Told the past partners that you found and felt comfortable telling now

Should You Go on Medications

32. Acknowledged your feelings and fears about starting or not starting on HIV medications right now

33. Questioned your doctor about the recommended treatment, including other options not involving medications

34. Completed the research checklist within the chapter, researching as much about different treatment methods as your mind would permit without overloading

35. Recognized that some people don't start taking medications unless lab results show their immune system weakening over time

36. Began taking HIV medications only because you felt comfortable doing so and not because of pressure from anyone else

Should You Keep Working or Go on Disability

37. Acknowledged your feelings and fears about being at work

38. Considered using work as a distraction right now if your job is low stress, or taking time off if your job is too stressful

39. Completed the time off checklist within chapter to understand what options you have to get time off

40. Recognized in which employer, state or provincial short-term disability plans you're enrolled, and made a claim for benefits if necessary

41. Analyzed whether you have a long-term disability that prevents you from working, and got assistance in making a claim for benefits

Should You Have Safe Sex or Not

42. Acknowledged your current interest in sex and the feelings associated with having it

43. Considered your idea of what safe or unsafe sex is for you and confirmed it with a knowledgeable professional like a physician, counselor or caseworker

44. Researched and recognized the serious emotional and physical risks that having unsafe sex might pose to your long term health and well being

45. Determined if at this time you are mentally and emotionally able to fully understand and accept the serious risks that having unsafe sex will bring into your life
46. Decided what sexual practices you will use for now and acknowledged the need to revisit this topic often in the future

Resource Examples

Honor Thy Children, Molly Fumia

Healing HIV: How to Rebuild Your Immune System, John D. Kaiser

National AIDS Manual Glossary, NAM Publications, www.nam.org.uk

Serenity: Support and Guidance for People with HIV, Their Families, Friends, and Caregivers, Paul Reed

National Pediatric & Family HIV Resource Center, www.pedhivaids.org
Look for: Guidelines and educational information about treatments for children with HIV

The Body Positive, www.thebody.com
Look for: Articles on how to choose a physician, how to tell your children and descriptions of state HIV notification laws

Aids Meds, www.aidsmeds.com
Look for: Detailed information about drug treatments, drug interactions and changes to protocols

Positive-Negative.Org, www.positive-negative.org
Look for: Support and guidance for when one partner is negative and one is positive

Canadian AIDS Society, www.cdnaids.ca
Look for: Age-appropriate guidelines for telling your children about HIV and AIDS

The Well Project, www.thewellproject.com
Look for: Guidelines for disclosing your status to people in your life, geared towards women

Chapter 3

Making Lifestyle Changes

At this point, you are putting a lot of the heavy stuff behind you. You are improving your coping techniques, using your support system and making important decisions that will help shape the future that you want for yourself. You are making great progress. I imagine that with each passing day, your situation is getting a little bit easier to handle and maybe a little less stressful, too. I told you that you had it in you. Keep up the good work.

It is time in this stage to move from your mental foundation to your physical one. So that your transition to living in peace with HIV may be successful, consider focusing some attention now on how your daily habits affect your health. Just as you can't build a good house without a solid foundation, you can't expect to have a peaceful existence with HIV without supporting your body in the process. Overall, the healthy habits discussed here are things you have probably known about for years but, for one reason or another, never quite put into practice. I'm certain you understand the increased importance for caring for your body now that HIV is part of your life. The following lifestyle topics are presented in a manner designed to get you thinking about what changes you might want to make for yourself. You may need to do additional reading and research for some topics to determine the specific programs or methods that will work for you.

When considering changes, remember that you built these habits up over a long time. Therefore, it may take a long time to change them as well. Changing everything at once would probably be too much for anyone, even if they haven't been through a recent crisis such as you have. You may be better off choosing a few areas to focus on in the short term, and then once you have made good progress, switch your attention to other areas. I do recommend that you create a plan now for changing each habit so you will be ready for action when the time comes to shift your focus from one area to another. Remember, there is no timeline for this stage of your journey, so take the right amount of time to make meaningful changes. These changes will become a permanent part of your foundation for peace and health.

Nutrition

There are a variety of opinions out there about what special nutritional needs people with HIV might have. Rather than join the debate, I think that for right now it is more important that you focus on adopting good overall nutritional habits as your foundation. There will be time down the line to fine tune your nutritional habits for any special HIV requirements.

We all know the old expression, "Garbage in, garbage out." It applies to nutrition as well. If you aren't eating food that provides fuel for your body and its cells, then you can't expect your body to do much for your health in return. It is that simple. Let me put this into context—if fast food or processed prepackaged meals are the center of your diet, you may be setting yourself up for big troubles ahead. Foods such as these that are heavy on fat, sodium, and additives and short on essential natural nutrients do zero for your quest to live a healthy life with HIV. Get the picture?

So what are good nutritional habits? There is no one answer. There have been hundreds of books written on the topic, all with different views on what type of diet is best for our bodies. At the core of almost every solid nutritional philosophy, however, is the idea that we should consume adequate amounts of carbohydrates, protein, and unsaturated fats on a daily basis. In addition, it is generally accepted that you should not skip meals, that you should eat several small meals a day instead of a few big ones, and that you should drink at least eight glasses of water daily to assist important bodily functions. That being said, deciding how much you should eat of which types of food is where the differing nutritional opinions come in. You will have to do some reading and research to decide what is right for yourself. You may decide instead to consult a nutritionist to assist you in developing a customized plan. Check out your local HIV/AIDS organizations to see if any of them offer this type of service. In the meantime, I have a few recommendations from my own experiences that I would like to share.

First off, try to eat food in a form as close as possible to its whole, natural state. The more a food is prepared and processed, the more nutritional value it loses along the way. For example, many frozen prepared foods will state that they contain vegetables, which might make you think you are getting some good nutrition. But often by the time they get to you, these vegetables have been so overcooked, chemically treated, or physically altered that it is very unlikely that much nutritional value is left in them. Fresh vegetables are always best, but frozen ones are fine as long as being frozen was all that was done to them. Just remember this rule of thumb: if you have a hard time recognizing a certain food in a finished product, then most likely your body will have trouble recognizing it, too.

Secondly, incorporate organic foods into your diet as much as possible. Organic foods are ones certified to have been grown or prepared without pesticides or chemicals, or in the case of meats, without antibiotics or growth hormones. These types of toxic substances are not good for anyone's body, but this is especially true for people with HIV, as we have a special need to support our internal functions and cells. You can find organic foods both at large grocery chains such as Whole Foods, Wild Oats, and Real Foods and at smaller local natural food markets. Organic foods can be expensive and difficult to come by in some areas, so they might not be within everyone's reach. If you can't afford or can't find organic foods, don't worry about it. You can still have great success in supporting your body by making wise nutritional choices at the regular grocery store. But if you are able to use organic products, give some strong consideration to doing so.

Lastly, after you eat, watch your body's reactions for a few hours. Are you experiencing any itching, stomach upset, or gas? If so, then you may have an internal food allergy of which you were unaware. Identifying these allergies and avoiding those foods that cause them is important to your health, because the energy your immune system wastes on fighting the allergy is taken away from its fight against HIV. I am certain that you want this energy directed towards supporting your immune system as opposed to attacking it.

You might be wondering how you can determine what food is causing your allergic reaction. Let me share a method that has worked for me. One day, I noticed that I experienced a fair amount of stomach upset and gas after eating a meal. I wrote down every ingredient included in that meal. Over the next week, I ate each one of those foods by itself, and then I watched my body's reaction over the next few hours to see if there was a problem. It turns out that I have an internal food allergy to spinach. Bummer. I really love spinach, but in the balance, the health of my immune system is far more important than my love of spinach.

Of course, change isn't always easy, especially when it comes to giving up foods we love. I have tempted fate a few times since my discovery by sneaking spinach into a meal, and each time I have paid the physical price for it. But worse than anything I experienced physically was the mental anguish of knowing I had made my immune system suffer, just because I lacked enough self control to stop. That kind of anguish seems like something you and I would want to avoid in our quest to live peacefully with HIV. I know I will in the future. Consider doing the same for yourself.

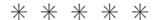

Vitamins and Supplements

Could the world of vitamins and supplements be any more confusing for consumers? Besides the sheer number of products on the market, the fact that so many claim to cure or improve the same conditions or ailments leaves my head spinning every time I walk into a vitamin store. Even when I decide that I should take a certain type of supplement, there are ten different brands from which to choose, each with different milligrams, different dosing schedules, and sometimes even different ingredients. How do I know which product is the right one for me to take? Does this one that costs twice as much as the one next to it mean that it is twice as good? Or are they just trying to rip me off? I get even more stressed because, having HIV, it seems doubly important that I find the right one to support my body. Calgon, take me away!

Okay, so maybe I was being a little overly dramatic, but I suspect you have no clue about which supplements to take to support your body now that you have HIV. This may be causing you a fair amount of stress. Relax. Help is on the way. Supplementation is one area of HIV treatment where there is an abundance of guidance. Plenty of research has emerged detailing which supplements can assist your immune system in fighting HIV. In fact, so many substances have shown good results that your wallet may empty and your medicine cabinet burst before you could buy all these helpful compounds. Therein lies the problem—how to pick and choose among the various options to design a supplement plan for you that is effective yet affordable.

One good source of guidance on this topic comes from buyers clubs. Buyers clubs are non-profit organizations formed to help people with HIV get high quality supplements at advantageous prices. These clubs usually ask for a small membership donation from you before you can take advantage of their services. The one I've used online, DAAIR, provides suggested supplementation plans at different levels, depending upon how much you can afford to spend, what type of medications you are taking, and what goals you are trying to achieve. I assembled my own current supplementation plan based primarily upon one of their recommendations, modified to reflect some reading I had done. When using a buyers club, be sure to place your order at least a few weeks before you will need the supplements. Most of these organizations are run by volunteers, so it may take a while for your order to be processed and shipped. It has sometimes taken my order two weeks to arrive, leaving me in the meantime to buy full-priced, lesser-grade supplements at the store. Definitely allow yourself plenty of lead time when ordering to avoid experiencing this type of financial pain. (Note: As of the publishing of this book, DAAIR had temporarily stopped its sale of supplements but planned to resume doing so at some point in 2004. During this time, however, all of DAAIR's good guidance about supplements is still kept current on their website, so don't hesitate to use it as a resource. In the meantime, I have switched to buying my supplements from the Houston Buyers Club, which has provided the same type of good service that DAAIR did.)

The good thing about supplements is that you can stop and start them easily, unlike medications. If you find that something doesn't work for you, then you can make adjustments and try something new. The bad thing about taking supplements is that you have to swallow more pills, which might be a psychological burden if you are already taking HIV medications several times a day. Some supplements are available in non-pill forms such as powder or crystals, in case you need a break from pill popping. Go ahead and look around online and in print to see what guidance exists to help you. In the meantime, let me tell you about three supplements that have worked well for me. Keep in mind that I am not endorsing these individual products in any way, and that you will have to do your own evaluation as to their safety and effectiveness for yourself.

A good multivitamin has been a key component in my supplementation plan, and I would recommend the same in yours. One study discovered that taking a multivitamin daily might reduce by 30% your chance of developing AIDS. The multivitamin that I have used, Super Blend by Super Nutrition, was formulated with HIV-positive people in mind and is carried by most buyers clubs and vitamin stores. Super Blend contains multitudes of vitamins, minerals, herbs and "superfoods" such as alfalfa leaves and spirulina. The recommended dosage is eight tablets a day, although I only use six a day to stretch each bottle further. Super Blend contains substantial amounts of many vitamins, minerals, herbs, and other nutritional compounds that you might have decided to buy separately. Therefore, you may save money by using it.

Immunocal® is the second supplement that you might want to consider. Without getting too technical, it is a milk protein isolate powder that helps increase gluthathione production in your body. Studies have identified gluthathione as extremely importantly to immune functions as well as being a contributor to long-term survival. Immunocal® may also help with reversing some HIV-related weight loss. I had a tough time finding Immunocal® anywhere but the Internet. Its price varies as much as 40% from website to website, so definitely search online for a bargain. When using Immunocal®, be sure not to mix it in a regular blender or dissolve it in hot water as both of these actions will destroy the chemical benefit of the powder.

The last supplement I want to mention is glutamine, sometimes listed as L-glutamine. For people with HIV, glutamine is somewhat of a wonder substance for all its benefits, especially its role in supporting T-cell creation and functioning. It also assists in detoxifying the liver, stimulating growth hormone for muscle development, and decreasing diarrhea. Pharmaceutical-grade glutamine powder is available from most buyers clubs and some vitamin stores. Glutamine is also available in capsule form, but you might have to swallow 15 to 20 capsules a day to get an effective dosage. I have found that capsules are handy for when you are traveling, especially if you don't want the stress of explaining to airport security or customs officers what this powdery white substance is in your bag!

One last thing to mention about supplements including herbs is the potential for adverse interaction with any medications that you might be taking, especially HIV medications. Be certain to ask your doctor about any known interactions when he or she prescribes a medication to you. You may also want to check with local HIV/AIDS service organizations for the latest information. A search of the Internet for guidance wouldn't hurt either. While ordering supplements from one online retailer, I noticed they had a link to a drug interaction listing for each supplement that they sell. You might want to check these websites for this type of information, even if you don't order anything. Hopefully, by using all these methods, you can get up-to-date information about known interactions and enjoy the best benefits of your supplements without worry.

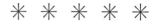

Exercise

We all know that some degree of exercise is necessary to maintain a healthy body. For some people, however, their fitness regime consists of walking from the front door to the car and back again. I don't think those two steps that you had to go up and down on your front porch are going to cut it in the long run.

There are two types of exercise to consider in your long-term survival plan. The first type is aerobic exercise, which is anything that elevates your heart rate for a sustained period of time. Aerobic activity uses oxygen and water to convert fat into energy, providing fuel for your body while also keeping off excess weight. This type of exercise improves your body circulation and assists your system in removing toxins left by medications you take and by foods you eat. It also keeps your heart healthy and improves your lung capacity, both of which will contribute to an overall feeling of increased energy. Be certain to drink plenty of water during aerobic activity, as this is when the greatest benefit of these internal body processes is received. Also, do your best to drink a fair amount of water throughout each day to keep these body processes functioning properly.

The other major type of exercise is anaerobic, which most of us associate with lifting weights. Anaerobic literally means without oxygen and is used to describe any exercise where your heart rate is not elevated for a sustained period of time. Instead of using oxygen and water to get energy, anaerobic exercise causes your body to pull energy from the food you eat and from energy stores in your muscles. The main goal of anaerobic weightlifting programs is to strengthen the muscles of the body in order to increase strength, reduce injuries, and support the body's organs and framework. Workout programs are usually designed to increase muscle strength, endurance, or size (or some combination thereof).

Why might you want to lift weights? Because statistics have shown that the majority of people that die of HIV-related illnesses don't die from the illness itself but rather from organ failure associated with a lack of lean body mass. Lean body mass is basically muscle, and HIV medications and the virus itself are thought to play roles in reducing this type of body mass over time. When you are fighting a major illness, your body will quickly use up fat stores, and then turn to lean body mass as a source of energy. Lean body mass takes longer than fat to breakdown, but once it is exhausted, your body starts to attack your organs in search of energy, causing organ failure. That's why working on your lean body mass may be important. Of course, you don't need to look like The Incredible Hulk to increase your chances of surviving a major illness. But you might consider working out regularly to at least keep the muscle that you already have and to possibly build more as an insurance policy. At any rate, if you decide not to workout or have to stop working out for a period of time, don't use this to project bad things for your future. Remember to stay focused on today, creating your own experience with HIV in the present.

There are hundreds of books to choose from when designing an exercise program for yourself. If you would like professional help, then consider hiring a personal trainer to create a program for you. Personal training can be expensive if you use it on a regular basis. But unless you need someone standing over you every time you exercise in order to be disciplined, consider hiring a trainer for just one or two sessions to design and demonstrate a workout program for you. You can use them again once every few months to update your program so that it matches your progress.

There are two more items to mention about exercise before I move on. First, glutamine can support your weight lifting efforts in addition to all its other great properties. Studies have shown that five grams of glutamine, taken on an empty stomach right before a workout, stimulates growth hormones and reduces the chance of post-workout illness. Extremely heavy or sustained workouts cause your immune system to dip, which is why you see so many professional athletics with colds and such. Glutamine has been shown in studies to reduce incidences of a post-workout illness by 50%. I have seen this play out for myself. I was lifting extremely heavy loads during my leg workouts. I noticed that the days after such workouts, I would experience flu-like symptoms such as some swollen glands, diarrhea, and general discomfort. Once I started using glutamine before my workouts, this problem completely disappeared. It was a nice confidence builder for me to have research studies I'd heard about actually translate into real-life benefits. Perhaps it may benefit you, too.

Second, I feel the need to mention steroids. In light of the news about the importance of lean body mass, there has been a growing movement advocating the use of steroids by people with HIV to build significant muscle mass. Steroids have some very negative connotations in society, mainly given to them by the media over the years. Rather than get into a lengthy discussion of the pros and cons of steroids, I think it is best to just bring up the option and then leave you to do your own research and decision making. In my own quest to increase lean body mass, I decided to try a non-steroid method for a year and then reevaluate my progress. After my year was up, I read a lot of research on steroids, talked with friends that have taken them, and discussed the matter with my doctor. While I have decided to not take them right now, I am keeping my mind open for the future. Before you begin any type of steroid program, be sure to do a fair amount of research about their use, including some on the potential severe negative health effects associated with it.

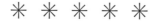

Stress Reduction

Stress affects our bodies in so many ways. It can cause or contribute to just about any pain, discomfort, or ailment you can possibly imagine. Think of the word disease in a different way:

dis-ease. Stress is *dis*-ease with something in your current situation. Stress-related ailments are signposts on the way to a major illness, which is how *dis*-ease ultimately shows up in the body. When you get used to having stress in your life, it is easy to lose sight of how damaging it has become to your health, both short and long term. Unfortunately, I found this out firsthand.

Two years after I was diagnosed, I switched from a routine, low-stress job to a more glamorous one with a higher stress potential to match its higher salary. After my first year on the job, a coworker died in a car accident. The stress of dealing with his death was too much for me, and I took two months off under a medical leave. I was certain that his death was the entire source of my stress. However, when I returned to work two months later all relaxed, the full stress of my job hit me like a tidal wave. Only then did I realize that when your stress level creeps up over time, you might barely notice the change, even though the cumulative stress could be doing some serious damage to your health. When I mentioned this to my doctor, she noted that my lab results had shown a slight decline in my immune system over the past year even though my medications hadn't changed. I felt very fortunate to get that wake-up call before I let stress ruin my health. And therein lies the beauty of recognizing when you are stressed—you can stop right there and do something to reduce your stress and protect your health. I call it talking yourself down off the ledge before you jump. In my case, it involved finding a new job that didn't cause me so much stress. But you will find your own way of dealing with the tensions in your life. You already have one breathing technique to help you. Let's discuss a few more methods that you can use for this purpose.

Some well-documented recent research revealed that 30 minutes of deep meditation each day could reverse the entire effect of a day's stress on the body. Wow! You couldn't ask for a cheaper or easier solution than that. But could it be true? I have become a believer. Since I began doing meditation every morning, I find that I am more focused, relaxed, and energetic throughout the day. It's also helped me to sleep better. When things go wrong during the day, they don't seem to bother me as much as they used to, creating even less stress than before.

Best of all, my health has never been better. Give meditation a try and see what it does for you.

When you hear the word *meditation,* you might be imagining someone sitting with their legs folded, chanting "oooohm" over and over again. I admit, that was my first thought, which I suspect is a result of watching too much television as a child. But as with everything else in your life, meditation can be made to fit your own style and needs. In my case, I put on headphones with relaxing music, lie down on the couch, and focus my mind on words such as *peace* and *good health*—both things I want in my life. Some people like to go outside, close their eyes, and use the sounds of nature to find a peaceful state. Whatever form it takes for you is not important, as long as the process helps your mind and body to take a break from the stresses of everyday life.

If you are one of those people who can't sit still long enough to meditate, maybe you should consider yoga. Yoga offers the same calming qualities as meditation, but it has you moving around instead of being still. Yoga requires you to get into different positions that help increase your flexibility, improve your circulation, and get the energy flowing inside your body. It is also an excellent way to develop your skill in using breathing for relaxation. There are many different styles of yoga to explore, so you can always keep it interesting by trying new movements and positions. Make no mistake about it, though, most yoga is a challenging workout. I would be surprised if you didn't find your muscles shaking and straining to hold some yoga positions. Yoga is usually taught in group classes at local yoga studios, community centers, or HIV/AIDS organizations. Due to yoga's growing popularity, many health clubs have also started offering group classes to their members. If you can't find a group class or would prefer to do it alone, there are private instructors out there as well as many instructional books and videos. I find yoga to be a nice balance to my weight lifting and other fitness activities.

As many of you probably already know, getting a massage is an excellent stress reduction technique. It has the added benefit of improving circulation, flushing out toxins, and loosening muscle constrictions. Usually, the biggest concern about massage is the cost. If you can't afford to pay full price for a massage, then check out some lower cost options. A local massage school may have a clinic where students give free or reduced price massages. Also, many local HIV/AIDS service organizations have lists of massage therapists that will massage you for free or at a reduced price because you have HIV.

Finally, if you find you need some additional help in reducing your stress, you may want to consult a counselor or therapist if you don't already have one. The bottom line is to find whatever methods or resources will help you to reduce your stress and live a more healthy life each day.

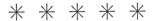

Sleep

My question to you is simple—do you get enough? If the answer is no, then you already know that you need to make some changes. Getting enough sleep each night is important on many levels. First of all, many of your body's regenerative processes occur while you are resting. For example, your kidneys wait until you are still before they start cleaning and rebalancing your blood. If you don't get enough sleep, you already start the day off with strikes against you in your goal to have good health. This is one reason you can never catch up on sleep. Trying to balance three hours of sleep one night with 10 hours the next doesn't cut it as far as your body is concerned. The damage has been done. Do your best to get a full night's sleep every night to give your body the greatest chance to be healthy every day.

Also, as we are all painfully aware, being short on sleep does nothing good for our moods and attitudes. Things that would have rolled off your back any other day suddenly become very irritating or a really big deal when you are sleep deprived. The resulting stress puts you in an even worse position physically than when you woke up that morning already behind in the health department. You know what I am trying to say.

If you are having trouble sleeping for some reason, try a few techniques that might help solve your problem before you consider using sleeping pills and the like. One is total body relaxation. Start at your toes and focus all your attention on relaxing them. Once they feel relaxed, move to your feet and ankles. Work your way up your body, relaxing one body part at a time. Most likely, before you even get near your head, you will be drifting off. If not, then continue focusing on relaxing your entire body all at once, imaging that you are floating. This should keep your mind free from the stressful thoughts that may be keeping you awake, giving you a better shot at falling asleep.

Warm milk just before bed is an old fashion remedy that really works for some people. Just as turkey does, milk contains tryptophan that helps make you sleepy. Warming the milk adds to the soothing effect, similar to tea. Just don't add anything with sugar or caffeine to the milk as you may be counteracting the relaxing effect you were trying to achieve.

My personal recommendation for light sleepers is to consider earplugs. Since I began using them, I am rarely kept awake or disturbed by noises, even when someone in the house is snoring loudly. Be sure to test that you can still hear things like smoke detectors and alarm clocks while you are using them, for your own safety. If you need background noise to drown out creaks and other sounds that keep you awake, consider using a fan in the room to provide this low-level background noise. I find this a particularly effective method in hotels, where we already face the challenge of trying to sleep well in a strange environment. Get creative in figuring ways to get a good night's sleep, and you'll be rewarded with not only improved health but possibly a better attitude as well.

✳ ✳ ✳ ✳ ✳

Smoking or Chewing

Most, if not all, of us would agree that smoking or chewing tobacco poses serious risks to one's health. We're all aware of the specific and well-documented risks. Therefore, if you do smoke or chew, then you have most likely acknowledged and accepted those risks. Now that you have HIV, however, consider revisiting the subject. In light of your new goal of a healthy, long-term peace with HIV, you should consider reviewing any habit that poses a substantial risk to your health.

If you do decide to quit smoking or chewing, acknowledge your current frame of mind to be certain that quitting wouldn't be too much for you to handle now. Definitely proceed with caution before creating a physical turmoil that might add to your mental one. In the balance, it might be better for you to continue smoking or chewing tobacco until your mind is in a less turbulent state. But if you decide to wait, revisit the idea of quitting often to see if your mental state has improved enough to support your attempt.

If you are finding it difficult to quit on your own, consider using a smoking cessation program. Some employers offer employees assistance programs of this type. Many health insurance plans also cover these programs. Your doctor may have some good advice about other effective methods including nicotine replacement programs. Support groups exist in some communities to help you make it through kicking this habit. The understanding and advice of someone who knows what you are going through can make all the difference in meeting your challenge, as I hope this book has shown you.

Drinking

Let me focus on the issues that consuming alcohol presents specifically for people with HIV. First, excessive or even moderate drinking can cause irreversible liver damage, which on its own can be fatal. This is because alcohol is metabolized in your liver. HIV medications are also metabolized in your liver. Given the high toxicity of many of these drugs, your liver may be sustaining damage from this process as well. Combine the effects on your liver of both drinking and HIV medications, and you may be putting your health at serious risk long term. If you are taking HIV medications, even a little alcohol can put additional strain on your liver. If you've had hepatitis or some other liver condition or have a history of such in your family, then the likelihood of liver trouble increases even more.

Certain HIV medications have the risk of causing pancreatitis, a condition in which the pancreas swells within the body, causing abdominal pain, shock, and sometimes collapse or even death. Studies have shown that using alcohol with certain HIV medications can significantly increase the likelihood of contracting this potentially fatal condition. Give some consideration as to whether you want to increase your odds of contracting pancreatitis by using alcohol.

Finally, drinking can sometimes lead to periods of impaired judgment. The risks you take during this time may have a direct effect on your health and the health of others. For example, you might have unprotected unsafe sex with another person, putting yourself at risk of catching another serious illness like hepatitis or getting re-infected with another strain of HIV. You might also end up infecting someone else with HIV. While I will discuss these health risks more in Chapter 5, you should understand for now that impaired judgment could lead to some serious health risks.

If you decide to quit drinking and need assistance in doing so, or if you think that you may be addicted to alcohol, consider using the same types of resources mentioned for those wanting to quit smoking. There are many people and organizations eager to help you, if you choose to ask them.

※　※　※　※　※

Recreational Drug Use

If you are taking HIV medications, I would be surprised if you wanted to put another drug into your body, even if just for fun! But being realistic, many people do just that. Similar to alcohol, the risks associated with impaired judgment and liver damage apply here as well. Unlike alcohol, however, which has standards for its production, you have no idea what is actually in most recreational drugs you might be tempted to buy and put into your body. Taking on this uncertainty is equal to spinning the wheel of chance with your health. You have no idea how the drug's contents will damage your body. Also, if you share a needle while injecting drugs, you could get re-infected with another more powerful strain of HIV.

If these types of risks are appealing or even glamorous to you, then perhaps the anger from your crisis mind or another event in your life has turned into hate and manifested itself in a self-destructive behavior. Then again, maybe your motivation is not quite that serious; perhaps it's just something you enjoyed doing for fun in the past. Regardless of why you want to do it, you need to recognize that the playing field has changed now that you have HIV. Living on the edge might be exciting for you, but if your goal is to live in peace with HIV, this type of risk may well prevent you from ever achieving that state of mind and health. It is your choice to make. If you do decide to stop using these drugs and need assistance, as with drinking, there are many resources out there to assist you.

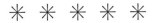

Caffeine

I can almost hear you right now. You are saying no junk food, no smoking, no drinking, and no recreational drug use. And now I'm suggesting that you stop using caffeine, the one vice that you have left? Maybe. Well, not really suggesting. More like presenting for your consideration.

As is the case with nicotine and sugar, caffeine is an addictive substance. It is a potent nervous system stimulant, but I probably don't need to tell you that if you ever consumed it to stay awake or to perk you up. Whether or not caffeine is bad for your health has never been completely agreed upon. Studies have show that for people with heart conditions, with peptic ulcers, or who are pregnant, caffeine consumption increases the risk of health complications. For the rest of us, its impact varies depending upon how much you consume and your genetic makeup. Some can consume a lot with no problems, while others have problems with any amount. Moderate to high consumption of caffeine has been associated with stomach upset, insomnia, vomiting, dehydration, headaches, and shakiness in some people. If you are experiencing any of these symptoms, try cutting back or eliminating caffeine to see if it helps. Also, caffeine can cause your body to lose water, so be sure to drink a few extra glasses of water daily if you are still consuming caffeine.

We all know that most coffees and teas have caffeine, but don't forget about other sources such as chocolate, sodas, and some brands of aspirin. Any pills that are marketed to keep you awake are jam-packed with it, as are most appetite suppressants. Many workout drinks and related products include caffeine as a stimulant. Also, so-called "energy drinks" get a lot of their energy from caffeine. If you decide to cut down or stop, start reading those labels to ensure that you meet your goals.

Also, caffeine does interact with some medications, so check with your doctor or search online to see if there is a potential issue for you. If you would like to cut down or stop consuming caffeine, search online for resources and methods that may assist you in your effort to kick this addiction.

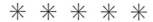

Helpful Exercises

You might have already considered making some lifestyle changes since hearing your diagnosis. Before you start, what do you already know that you need to change in these areas? Take a moment to write those changes down in your journal as a reference point for when you are considering each habit in more detail later.

To assist you in fitting these changes into your busy life, stop now and create a one-week schedule grid in your journal. Across the top of the page, make the following columns: *Time, Monday, Tuesday, Wednesday, Thursday, Friday, Saturday,* and *Sunday.* In the *Time* column, record each hour of the day starting with 7:00 a.m. and going through 6:00 a.m. the next day. I thought it would be easiest for you to start scheduling your day with what you do each morning, and then work forward through your day until you go to sleep each night.

Using this grid, record every time commitment that you have during an average week, and be realistic about what activities that you actually do. Yeah, you thought about going to the gym four times last week, but only count the actual times that you made it inside the building and exercised! Don't forget things like sleeping, eating, and watching television. You will be using this schedule many times in the exercises ahead to help you to create your plan for healthy changes to your life. If possible, use different colored inks when you make any additions or changes to this schedule. That will help you to keep track of what your new plan looks like overall.

Nutrition

How would you describe your diet now? What are the main types of food that you eat each day? How many meals do you have each day and when do you eat them? Do you eat a lot of fast food or prepackaged meals? What do you eat for snacks?

Your answers should give you a general idea of what your current approach to nutrition is, no matter how bad it might sound. How many calories do you think that you eat each day? Don't forget to include beverages such as juice and milk in your count. Find a calorie chart in a book or online to help out with your calculations. How many glasses of water do you drink each day? How much energy do you have after a meal? Do you tend to get sleepy after you eat or crash a few hours later?

There is one more calculation to do before you are finished with your initial assessment. How many calories do you need to eat each day? A common method for arriving at this number uses your body weight and your level of physical activity. Use the simple formulas and chart below to determine how many calories you need in order to maintain your current weight and how many you would need to eat to reach your ideal body weight. Record the results of your calculations in your journal. When picking your ideal weight, focus on what you would like to weigh in two or three months rather than the perfect weight for you. You can adjust this ideal weight downward again after you achieve this first weight goal. A side note: if math is not your thing and you already know you want professional help in designing a nutrition plan, then consider letting a nutritionist do the math for you.

Current Weight X Calories Per Pound (from below) = Current Calories
Ideal Weight X Calories Per Pound (from below) = Ideal Calories

10 calories per pound = inactive to slightly active
12 calories per pound = somewhat to moderately active
15 calories per pound = moderately to very active
18 calories per pound = extremely active

The basic idea is that to maintain your current body weight or reach your ideal weight, you need to eat the total number of calories you calculated for each one above. Sounds simple enough, yes? Now comes the confusing part—deciding where those calories should come from.

Unfortunately, because there are so many approaches, I can't give you guidance here that is tailored to your individual needs. You will have to research and design a plan on your own. This could involve reading some of those books you've seen or heard about. You should definitely consider doing searches on the Internet using the keywords *HIV* and *nutrition* as there is a lot of guidance online for people with HIV. Your local HIV/AIDS service organization may already have some materials to share with you on the topic. If you would like some professional help, consider consulting a nutritionist either through your health plan or on your own. With all the information you have gathered from the exercises and calculations above, you've made a great start on creating a healthy nutrition plan for yourself. Use your journal now to write down your ideas of how to create the plan, as well as to take notes while searching on the Internet or consulting people by telephone.

Supplements

What supplements are you already taking? By supplements, I mean vitamins, minerals, herbal remedies, and workout products. How much do you spend each month on supplements? Make a list in your journal of these supplements, and estimate the monthly cost of each. You might be surprised at the total that you spend.

Now you have a clear picture of where you are at currently. So where do you go from here? As with nutrition, your supplement needs are unique to your own body and health, so you will have to design your own approach that fits your life. There is a great deal of guidance out there about which supplements that HIV people can use to support their bodies. You will find this guidance in the same places as the nutritional information from above. Also, as I mentioned earlier, check into local and national buyers clubs, some of which are on the Internet. Most of these clubs have suggested supplementation plans that vary depending upon your budget, the medications you're taking, and your goals for taking supplements. You already know how much you are spending on supplements, so check your budget to see if you can increase it. Over time, you can add or drop supplements to fine-tune your plan to meet your needs and budget. Take some time now to start creating your plan in your journal. Make notes from your online searches or calculations about how much that you can spend each month on supplements.

Exercise

Easy first question—what type of exercise do you do right now? Be specific about what each activity is, how long it lasts, and how many times that you do it in an average week.

As you may recall, there are two main types of exercise, aerobic and anaerobic. To get the maximum cardiovascular benefits from aerobic exercise, you need to do it continuously for at least 30 minutes. Doing aerobic exercise three or four times a week is recommended for most people. Go back to the exercise list you just made and label everything that qualifies as aerobic activity.

Anaerobic exercise may involve moments of elevated heart rate but not for a sustained period. Weight lifting is the one activity that most people with HIV focus on in an effort to build up their lean body mass, making their bodies stronger and better able to fight off a serious illness. Go back to your list and label every exercise that qualifies as anaerobic.

Next you need to decide what your goals are for exercising. Are you trying to lose weight, improve your circulation, build your muscles to add lean body mass, or keep your heart healthy? Maybe you are after a combination of these goals with a few others thrown in. Write your goals down now to use later in designing an exercise plan that meets them.

Now you are ready to put together an exercise plan for yourself. As is the case with nutrition, there are many books on the subject, each with a slightly different approach. Definitely search online using keywords like *exercise, fitness,* and *muscle.* Consider hiring a personal trainer to design a program for you. Check with your local HIV/AIDS service organization to see if they provide this type of service, have exercise guidance, or can make a referral to a personal trainer or health club that will give you a reduced price. Use your journal to start designing your exercise plan, to make notes from your online research, or to organize your thoughts about exercise. Once you have the plan put together, go back to your weekly schedule and put in your exercise times.

Stress Reduction

Stress is a part of life. At least that is what you always hear. How is stress a part of your life? Where does your stress come from? Is it from your work, your home life, or somewhere else? Make a list of what causes you to experience stress in your life. For each item in your list, record how the stress from it affects you mentally, physically, and emotionally. When identifying a source of stress, be as specific as you can about what events, actions, or circumstances associated with that source are causing the stress.

Sometimes the stress in our lives increases so slowly that we don't realize how much we have taken on, yet our body is fully aware of all the damage that this stress is inflicting. Do you do anything now to reduce your stress? What else can you do to reduce the stress in your life, now that you have recognized where it comes from and what it does to you? Take a few moments and think about what actions that you could take, the new ways that you could think, or the changes you could make that would reduce the sources of your stress in your life. Use your journal to record your thoughts and ideas.

Even though your efforts to reduce stress at the source hopefully will pay off, some stress is likely to remain. How can you deal with it effectively? You already know about some good breathing techniques from Chapter 1. Don't forget to consider meditation, yoga, massage, qigong, chiropractic adjustments, and acupuncture, just to name a few other methods. Use your journal now to come up with a plan for reducing or eliminating the effects of stress on your mind, body and spirit. And don't forget to add this time to your weekly schedule. The peace that you will find from reducing stress is worth every minute of your time that you have invested.

Sleep

Ah, sleep. Most of us probably think of sleep as a luxury. It's something we all want but tend to sacrifice in order to make time for things we think of as necessities in life, such as work, family, and friends. How much sleep do you get on an average night? Is it enough? Does the amount vary significantly from night to night? How do you feel when you wake up each morning? If you don't get enough sleep or don't sleep well, why do you think that is?

So maybe you already know that sleep is a problem for you. The general rule is that you should get at least eight hours each night. This varies from person to person, but I'll bet you know how much is enough for you to feel good and rested. If you are having trouble sleeping, try to understand why. Is it that your mind won't be quiet? Are there noises that keep you awake? Are you just not tired when you climb into bed? Take some time here to try and figure out the source of your problem.

Some solutions others have used for sleeping problems include doing breathing exercises to relax, using earplugs to block out noise, or getting enough exercise during the day to tire oneself out. As a last resort, there are always sleeping pills, but you definitely don't want to take any more drugs than you have to at this point in your life. Reflect on what you have written in your journal so far in this section. What changes will you make to get enough sleep each night? Make a plan now and add your new sleeping hours to your weekly schedule. It is time to put more luxury into your life.

Smoking or Chewing

Do you smoke cigarettes? Do you smoke tobacco using a pipe? Do you chew tobacco? How much do you smoke or chew each day or each week? How long have you had this habit? Be honest as this is for your own benefit.

Now you should have a clear picture of your smoking or chewing habit. So why do you do it? Every action that we take in life has a payoff for us, even if it appears to be a negative one. What does smoking or chewing give you? Why do you enjoy it?

So you see why smoking or chewing has worked for you in the past. Now that you have HIV, consider reviewing this payoff in light of your new concerns for your long-term health. Does it still make sense for you to continue a habit you know will cause you health problems later? Only you can answer that question.

Have you ever tried to quit before? If so, how long did it last? Why did you start smoking or chewing again? Some of you may even have started again when you got your diagnosis! Take a moment to record your history with this habit.

You now understand how you have done it and why you have done it. Now, the question is, do you want to keep doing it or quit? If you would like to quit, there are many resources out there to support your effort. Your employer may provide or pay for a smoking cessation program. Your doctor can pre-scribe a nicotine patch to help ease you off of it. There are also support groups out there that can help. Your local HIV/AIDS service organization may be of assistance in finding some of these resources. You can also check online under the keywords *quit smoking* or *smoking cessation*. If you want to quit, take a moment here to come up with a plan. You can also your jour-nal to record any notes from searching the Internet or making calls to find resources to help you.

Drinking

You may have had the urge to get good and drunk a few times since your diagnosis. Heck, maybe even you did it. We all have to find a way to cope in the short term. But let's focus on your long-term habit instead. How much alcohol do you drink each day or each week? Does how much you drink vary greatly from day to day? How long have you been drinking? What do you enjoy about it? What does it give you?

Let's switch gears for a moment. What medications are you currently taking? Have you ever had hepatitis or some other type of liver condition? Is there a history of liver trouble in your family?

Combine the effects on your liver of both alcohol and HIV medications, and your health may be in some serious trouble. You should keep in mind that even small amounts of alcohol might cause liver damage. If you've had any illness that affected your liver or have a family history of such, then the likelihood of trouble increases even more. There are other HIV-related dangers (such as pancreatitis) surrounding drinking.

You will have to make your own decision about whether or not to keep drinking. If you would like to quit, there are resources out there to assist you. Your employer may have an employee assistance plan that includes help to quit drinking, or you could consider enlisting the help of a therapist. There are support groups out there as well as entire community service organizations devoted to assisting you in stopping. Your local HIV/AIDS service organization may be able to refer you to some of these resources. Consider doing an online search using keywords like *alcohol dependency, stop drinking,* and *clean and sober.* Start your plan here today. Take some time to write down what you would like to change. Also use your journal to make notes while you research the support options available for you in your community.

Recreational Drug Use

What is a recreational drug? Basically, it is any drug or chemical that you put in your body for "fun" instead of for medical purposes. You might swallow, inhale, or inject it. What recreational drugs do you use? How often do you use them? How much do you use at one time? How do you feel after using each type? How do you feel the day after using a drug?

If you have started taking HIV medications, why would you want to put any other drugs in your body unless absolutely necessary? What is your motivation for taking recreational drugs? What is the payoff that you get from doing it? Is it something that you find exciting to do? Does it help you to escape?

If you were honest in answering the above questions, at least you understand why you take recreational drugs. If you are interested in quitting, there are many resources out there to support you. Just as there are for drinking, there are support groups, employer assistance plans, therapists, and community organizations to assist you in your effort. Your local HIV/AIDS service organization should be able to direct you to resources in your area. Doing an online search using keywords like *drug dependency, drug addiction,* and *drug recovery* might provide some useful information. Use your journal to start planning how you will quit as well as to take notes about the resources that you discover are available to you in your community.

Caffeine

Caffeine deserves some consideration on its own because of its potential health effects and widespread use. How much caffeine do you consume each day? Think in terms of cups of coffee or cans of soda. What are the sources of your caffeine? Why do you consume it? Is it for the taste of the product that it is in or to give you a boost of energy?

You may be consuming a lot more caffeine than you think since some sources of caffeine are not well known. Let's do a little math in your journal to give you a better idea of how many milligrams that you take ingest in an average day. Again, if math isn't your thing, at least come up with a realistic estimate of your daily caffeine consumption by looking at the items listed below.

When adding up your caffeine consumption, don't forget to increase the number of units to reflect how many ounces you actually take in. For examples, sodas come in sizes that start at 12 ounces and go up to over 100 ounces! That means if you drink one of those big ones, you may have consumed more than 16 units for just that one beverage alone. That translates into more than 600 mg of caffeine. Don't worry if your math isn't perfect here, as you are just trying to get a rough idea of how much caffeine that you are consuming each day.

Product/Substance (One Unit)	Milligrams of Caffeine per Unit
Coffee, 6-ounce cup	130 mg
Tea, 6-ounce cup	55 mg
Soda, 6-ounce cup	50 mg
Cocoa, 1-ounce dry	45 mg
Diet pill, one capsule	200 mg
No-sleep pill, one tablet	150 mg
Pain relievers (some), one tablet	50 mg
Energy drinks (some), 8-ounce cup	130 mg

So what was your grand total? Were you surprised at how high the number was? A daily intake of 500 mg or more of caffeine is considered high and puts you at the greatest risk of developing negative health effects from its use. Consuming 250-500 mg a day is considered a moderate risk and 100-250 mg a day a low risk. How caffeine affects you individually depends upon your genetics and your other lifestyle habits to some degree.

Now that you know how much caffeine you consume and what the potential risks are, decide for yourself if you should cut back or stop all together. If your goal is to live in peace with HIV, then consider the potential effect of daily caffeine use on your health. I have found the most information about caffeine online, though I am certain there are books out there, too. Search online by using keywords like *caffeine, caffeine addiction,* and *caffeine health*. If you already know that you want to cut back or quit, then start your plan now. Use your journal to identify the changes that you are going to make and to record any notes from your research about caffeine.

Chapter 3 Checklist

Complete the following checklist in your journal before moving on to Chapter 4. These lifestyle changes are important for building your physical foundation, which gives your body every chance to be healthy each day. You will need to complete each step below before you reach the next stage in Chapter 5. Number a page in your journal from 1 to 54, and record the date that you complete each step.

First Steps:

1. Acknowledged changes in your lifestyle habits that you already know that you need to make
2. Created weekly schedule showing all activities you complete during an average week

Nutrition

3. Acknowledged what your current eating habits are, such as the types of foods that you eat and when you eat them
4. Estimated how many calories you eat each day and acknowledged how you feel after meals

5. Calculated how many calories you should be eating to maintain your current weight and to attain your ideal weight
6. Researched different nutritional approaches and considered possibility of using a nutritionist
7. Created and began using a nutritional plan that supports your body's needs and overall health

Supplements

8. Identified what supplements you are already taking and how much they cost you monthly
9. Researched supplement guidance for people with HIV by going online, using books, or contacting your local HIV/AIDS service organization for assistance
10. Considered using a buyers club to research supplementation plans and to purchase supplements
11. Created and began using a supplementation plan that meets your physical needs as well as your budget

Exercise

12. Identified what exercise activities you already do, how often you do them, and for how long you do them each time
13. Identified whether each activity that you do is aerobic or anaerobic
14. Determined your desired health goals for exercising
15. Researched different fitness approaches by searching online, using books, or contacting your local HIV/AIDS service organization or a personal trainer
16. Created and began to follow an exercise program that meets your desired health goals
17. Put time for exercise into your weekly schedule created in this chapter

Stress Reduction

18. Identified the sources of stress in your life and how that stress affects your mind, body, and spirit

19. Recognized ways to reduce this stress at the source and took steps to do so
20. Began to reduce the remaining stress by using one or more stress reduction methods on a daily basis, including breath work, meditation, yoga, and massage
21. Created and began using a plan for reducing or eliminating the effects of stress on your mind, body, and spirit
22. Put daily time for stress reduction activities into your weekly schedule created in this chapter

Sleep

23. Identified how much sleep you get each night, if it is enough sleep for you, and how you feel when you wake up
24. Recognized that your body needs adequate sleep every night to fully regenerate after each day's wear and tear
25. Accepted that you can never make up for lost sleep and its negative effect on your body and health
26. Identified any problems that you have sleeping and found solutions to address each one
27. Created and are following a plan to get sufficient sleep for your body and health each night
28. Put daily time for sleep into your weekly schedule created in this chapter

Smoking or Chewing

29. Acknowledged that you have a smoking or chewing habit, including how much and how often
30. Recognized what this habit gives you and why you enjoy it
31. Accepted that smoking or chewing is bad for your health, especially now that you have HIV
32. Recorded the history of your habit, including any times that you tried to quit and how long you were successful
33. Researched resources to assist you in quitting this habit, if you decided to quit

34. Created and began following a plan to quit smoking to avoid its negative effects on your health, if you decided to quit

Drinking

35. Acknowledged that you drink alcoholic beverages, including how much and how often
36. Identified any medications that you are taking, any liver conditions that you have had and any family history of liver problems
37. Accepted that both alcohol use and toxic medications, like most HIV drugs, can cause liver damage, especially when used together
38. Acknowledged the increased risk of pancreatitis associated with HIV drug use and drinking alcohol
39. Acknowledged that drinking alcohol can cause impaired judgment, possibly causing you to take risks that result in your re-infection with HIV or catching other illnesses
40. Researched resources to assist you in quitting this habit, if you decided to quit
41. Created and began following a plan to quit drinking to avoid its negative effects on your health, if you decided to quit

Recreational Drug Use

42. Acknowledged what recreational drugs that you use, how much you take at one time, and how often you do it
43. Accepted that recreational drugs are not regulated and could contain anything in any amount, which may cause your body and health unpredictable damage now that you have HIV
44. Recognized the reasons why that you take recreational drugs, including any self-destructive urges
45. Acknowledged that recreational drug use can cause impaired judgment, possibly causing you to take risks that result in your re-infection with HIV or catching other illnesses

46. Researched resources to assist you in quitting this habit, if you decided to quit
47. Created and began following a plan to quit using recreational drugs to avoid their negative effects on your health, if you decided to quit

Caffeine

48. Analyzed your idea of how much caffeine you consume each day, what sources you get it from, and what it does for you
49. Calculated how much caffeine you may actually be consuming each day, using the chart for guidance
50. Acknowledged that consumption of more than 100 mg a day presents some health risks, with consumption of 500 mg or more each day presenting the greatest risks
51. Recognized the possible health risks from caffeine use include birth defects, certain cancers, stomach ulcers, and hypertension
52. Recognized that symptoms like headache, tremors, insomnia, stomach upset, dehydration, depression, and anxiety have been associated with its use
53. Researched online and through books about the effects of caffeine on the body and health
54. Created and put into place a plan to reduce or eliminate caffeine consumption, if you decide to cut back or stop

Resource Examples

The Glucose Revolution, Thomas M.S. Wolever, et al

Built to Survive, Michael Mooney, Nelson Vergel

Body for Life: 12 Weeks to Mental and Physical Strength, Bill Phillips

Conscious Breathing: Breathwork for Health, Stress Release and Personal Mastery, Gay Hendricks

Your Body's Many Cries for Water : You Are Not Sick, You Are Thirsty, Fereydoon Batmanghelidj

Meditations for Enhancing Your Immune System, Bernie S. Siegel

Comparative Guide for Nutritional Supplements, Lyle MacWilliam

Nutrition and HIV: A New Model for Treatment, Mary Romeyn

50 Ways to Build Muscle Fast, Dave Tuttle

The Relaxation & Stress Reduction Workbook, Martha Davis, et al

Deep Sleep: Complete Rest for Health, Vitality and Longevity, John R. Harvey

Yoga for Stress Relief, Swami Shivapremananda

Super Healing Foods, Frances Sheridan Goulart

American Lung Association 7 Steps for a Smoke-Free Life, Edwin B. Fisher

Conquering Caffeine Dependence: Natural Approaches to Reducing Caffeine Intake, Mike Fillon

How to Quit Drinking without AA: A Complete Self-Help Guide, Jerry Dorsman

Eating Positive: A Nutrition Guide and Recipe Book for People with HIV/AIDS, Jeffrey T. Huber, Ph.D. and Kris Riddlesperger

Mediation for Dummies ®, Stephan Bodian

Cooking for Life: A Guide to Nutrition and Food Safety for the HIV-Positive Community, Robert H. Lehmann

Project Inform, www.projinf.org
Look for: Excellent guidance on drug interactions, including dangers of mixing recreational drugs or alcohol with HIV medications

DAAIR, www.daair.org
Look for: Guidance on supplementation plans that meet your goals and budget

Houston Buyers Club, www.houstonbuyersclub.com
Look for: Low-priced high quality supplements available to people with HIV or AIDS

HIV Resources, www.hivresources.com
Look for: Nutritional guidance including email newsletter and book recommendations

Think Muscle, www.thinkmuscle.com
Look for: Articles, newsletter and message boards about building muscle mass

The Vitamin Shoppe, www.vitaminshoppe.com
Look for: Online health guide containing drug interaction list for nutrients and herbs that it sells

The Body Positive, www.thebody.com
Look for: Articles about stress reduction methods and ways to fight depression

Association of Nutrition Service Agencies, www.aidsnutrition.org
Look for: Fact sheets for nutritionally treating side effects and other unpleasant conditions

Chapter 4

Using Federal, State and Community Resources

Throughout this book, I have made reference to using federal, state, provincial, and community resources to help you to do things like get disability benefits, find out the latest on treatment options, or enjoy the benefits of a free massage. Now it is time to give you more detailed information about what resources exist and whether or not you may qualify to use them. Knowing and using the resources available to you will definitely help you build that solid foundation you are seeking. The information provided below for federal and state programs is geared towards people living in the U.S. If you live in another country, check with your federal, state, or provincial government to see what similar programs are available to you.

After I run you through the different types of programs, you will need to do some searching on your own to find the local HIV/AIDS service organizations that can best assist you. The fantastic thing about most HIV/AIDS service organizations is that because their mission is to serve people in need, they will freely refer you to other community resources to help you get all the assistance you are seeking.

One good way to find local HIV/AIDS service organizations is to ask your doctor about them. You could also try surfing the Internet or consulting your phone book for listings. During your search, don't forget to check out community resources that serve the general population by providing things like food, housing, job training, and such. Also keep in mind that most major religions run charitable service organizations, including ones focused on helping people with HIV/AIDS. As you will see, the resources are out there, just waiting for you to raise your hand and ask for help.

Federal Programs

There are no U.S. federal programs designed specifically for people with HIV/AIDS. Instead, federal funds are directed to state and local HIV/AIDS service organizations to help them provide services to people living with HIV or AIDS. However, people with HIV or AIDS commonly access two general federal programs, Social Security and Medicare.

Social Security has two programs within it: Social Security Disability Income (SSDI) and Supplemental Security Income (SSI). SSDI is available only to people that have paid taxes into the Social Security system, usually through wages deductions. SSI does not require that you have paid taxes and is based upon your income level and the amount of financial resources you have. You can receive both benefits at the same time if you meet each program's eligibility requirements.

To qualify for either program, you have to receive an official disability determination from the Social Security Administration (SSA). As I mentioned in Chapter 2, receiving this determination has become increasingly difficult over time as medical advances have greatly improved the health and daily functioning of people with HIV. I received this information straight from the source, a friend whose job at the SSA was to make these determinations. This doesn't mean that you shouldn't apply for these benefits, but definitely be aware that having HIV while being otherwise healthy is probably not enough for you to receive the required disabled determination. If the SSA does determine you to be disabled, you may automatically qualify for benefits from other programs, including private ones, without having to provide additional evidence of your disability.

Medicare, which you may think of as health insurance for the retired, also provides health insurance for people that are receiving SSDI benefits. However, keep in mind that Medicare benefits don't kick in until 24 months after you receive your first SSDI benefit check. You have to pay a monthly premium for Medicare coverage, though some states have programs that will pay this premium for you if you qualify. Also, Medicare doesn't provide coverage for prescription drugs, though that may be changing soon. As I will discuss below, some states have programs that provide HIV medications for people with low income and no or limited drug coverage.

Medicare has undergone many changes in recent years, including adding HMOs to their system. Some of these HMOs had full prescription drug coverage at one time, but now many have eliminated this coverage or capped it at a very low annual amount. If you still have insurance through your employer, either as an active employee or through COBRA, it may be smarter for you to hold onto that insurance instead. I will discuss insurance more in Chapter 6. For now, contact your local HIV/AIDS service organization for assistance in making this analysis as well for up-to-date information about these and other federal programs. Also, the SSA has a free publication geared towards people with HIV/AIDS that describes the benefits available, eligibility requirements and how to file a claim.

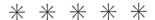

State Programs

The primary state programs that people with HIV access are for health insurance, drug coverage, and disability benefits. Medicaid (health insurance primarily for low-income individuals) is a federal program that is administered by each state. Each state receives a block of federal funding which it then combines with its own funds to provide this medical insurance to state residents that qualify. Eligibility requirements, items covered, and payment amounts vary from state to state. If you qualified for federal SSI benefits, then most states automatically make you eligible for Medicaid because of your low income level. In some states, SSI recipients may also qualify for food stamps and additional supplemental income benefits. In addition, some states have programs that will help pay your Medicaid or other insurance premiums. Be sure to check with your local HIV/AIDS service organization for details about these and other insurance programs.

For HIV-positive people with low incomes and limited or no prescription drug coverage, most states offer a program that will provide HIV/AIDS medications for free or a low co-pay. This federally supported program is called the AIDS Drug Assistance Program (ADAP) in most states, though some states have their own unique name for it. The eligibility and types of medications covered vary from state to state. Unfortunately, due to the overwhelming need for these drugs, many state programs have had to start waiting lists for people wanting to enroll. Don't let this discourage you, however, from applying for coverage if you meet the eligibility requirements in your state. Even if you end up on a waiting list, you will at least have the comfort of knowing you're in line to get the medications just as soon as they become available to you. Check with your local HIV/AIDS service organization for the inside scoop on these programs and assistance in applying. Keep in mind that ADAPs normally only cover HIV/AIDS medications. You will still be on your own for any other prescriptions you might have. Your local HIV/AIDS organization may be able to tell you of other programs that can help you to get coverage for these other medications.

A few states have their own state-run short-term disability program that you may be able to access. These programs are normally funded by premiums deducted as a tax from your paycheck. If your employer also has a short-term disability program, you may have elected to pay premiums to that plan instead, thereby opting out of the state plan. Many people choose to do this because employer plans tend to have more generous benefits than those from the state. If you do opt out of the state plan, you will only be able to receive short-term disability benefits from your employer. Check with your employer plan's administrator to see what options are available to you. In addition, your state may have other programs that could assist you in meeting your needs during your time of disability. For example, if you didn't pay Social Security tax on your wages, you may have paid premiums to a state retirement system like PERS instead. You may be able to get disability benefits from this program as well. Contact your local HIV/AIDS service organization to get additional information on state programs and for assistance in filing claims.

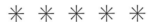

Local HIV/AIDS Service Organizations

Depending upon where you live, there may be a lot of HIV/AIDS service organizations or virtually none. In general, the bigger a city's population, the more service organizations it has. Still, there are few smaller cities out there that buck the trend. Regardless of where you live, definitely do a diligent search before you give up and think there's nothing out there to help you. And when you are searching online, don't forget to check the links page of any HIV/AIDS service organization website that you come across. Their site may include links to similar service organizations in your local area.

So what types of services do these organizations usually provide? You might be surprised at the depth of the answer. Here is a partial listing of the services I've seen offered for free or at a reduced price: counseling, HIV medications, health insurance premium payments, assistance in filing benefit claims, legal advice, housing vouchers, food vouchers, home meal delivery, community resource guidebooks, haircuts, massages, energy work, chiropractic adjustments, nutritional counseling, Internet access, computers, yoga classes, and gym memberships. In addition, some organizations offer peer advocacy, a service similar to this book where someone who has experience living with HIV offers you guidance and support. Another service I have seen is case management, a situation where a well-connected person takes charge of helping you get everything you need from community resources.

The primary requirement for accessing most of these services is having proof of your HIV or AIDS diagnosis. In my volunteer work in the benefits area, I have seen this range from an official doctor's letter on letterhead to a short note scribbled on a prescription pad. A copy of your lab results showing HIV present in your blood is sometimes also acceptable as long as your name is printed on it. Doctors are accustomed to providing a diagnosis letter when needed, so don't be afraid to ask for one. You will only have to do it once if you keep a copy of the letter for future use. Many times, the HIV/AIDS service organization that you are trying to use will help you get this letter if you don't already have it.

Most services are available to you regardless of how much income you have. A few programs, however, do have upper income limits in order for you to qualify. If you have to prove your income, be prepared to provide your last income tax form. If your income has dropped significantly from the amount on your income tax form, a recent pay stub might be a better indication for you to show them. Of course, if you are unemployed or collecting disability, you may already qualify.

Some organizations may ask you to prove that you are a local resident before you can access certain services. Normally this process involves showing a utility bill with your name and address on it. This could be your telephone, electric, or cable bill, for example. I have only seen one organization with this requirement, but it is always good to check. Many organizations have consciously decided not to make residency a requirement for their services, recognizing that it may be difficult for homeless or transient persons and undocumented residents to provide sufficient proof.

One last thing to mention about using these organizations is confidentiality. As I will discuss in Chapter 5, there are laws prohibiting the disclosure of your medical information without your authorization. I have never heard of an organization breaching this confidentiality, but it may happen in isolated incidences. Get their confidentiality policy in writing, discuss it with them if you have concerns, and hold onto the policy in case you need to file a legal complaint later. That being said, you may soon come to realize that most of the people whom work and volunteer at these organizations are passionately interested in helping you meet your needs on your journey to living in peace with HIV. Consider opening your heart to the help that is available.

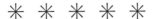

Helpful Exercises

If you live in the U.S., go ahead and start your work in this chapter with the Federal Programs section below. If you live in another country, use your journal now to make notes during your search for federal, state, and provincial resources of a similar nature. Your doctor or your local health department or ministry may be a good place to start your search. In the exercises below, skip down to the Local HIV/AIDS Service Organizations section for help in locating these types of organizations in your area.

Federal Programs

Social Security and Medicare are the two federal programs usually accessed by people with HIV. Have you ever received benefits from these programs before? For what reasons did you receive them?

Many programs require that you have paid certain taxes in order to get benefits. Has Social Security tax been deducted from your paycheck in the past? If not, was another type of retirement tax deducted instead, such as PERS? Have your received a statement from the Social Security Administration that shows your SS tax paid and potential benefits? Have you received the same statement from PERS, if applicable?

Even if you don't need to access these programs now, it is still a good exercise to find out the type and dollar amount of these benefits that you might be entitled to if disabled. But let me ask, do you have a disability now that prevents you from working? What is it? Is it HIV-related? Would your medical records support your disability claim? How?

To receive benefits from Social Security or Medicare, you must first receive a disability determination from the Social Security Administration (SSA). Getting this disability determination for having HIV is difficult to do if you are otherwise healthy. The SSA has put out a brochure specifically about this issue to both offer guidance and to inform you how to file a claim for benefits. Contact the SSA for a copy or visit their website at www.ssa.gov.

Now that you have a few more details, do you think you might be eligible for any federal programs? Which ones? Will you file a claim? Whom will you contact to follow up? Your local HIV/AIDS service organization may be able to provide you assistance in determining what benefits you may be eligible for and filing the appropriate claim. Take some time now to create your plan of action in your journal, and then go out and get the benefits that you need right now.

State Programs

Similar to the federal programs, some states have health insurance plans that people with HIV access, including Medicaid. Have you ever claimed Medicaid or other types of state health insurance benefits? What was the reason? Are you still receiving state health insurance benefits today?

Medicaid eligibility requirements and benefits vary from state to state. Check with your state health office or contact your local HIV/AIDS service organization for more information and assistance in applying for Medicaid and other state health insurance benefits.

A few states have public short-term disability plans. Have you claimed state disability benefits before, excluding worker's compensation benefits? What was the reason? Are you still receiving state disability benefits today?

Your employer might have a short-term disability plan that you can access as well. However, you can only claim benefits from the one plan to which you paid premiums, so keep that in mind when you go to file a claim. Check with your employer plan's administrator, your state insurance office or your local HIV/AIDS service organization for more information and assistance in filing a claim. Be sure to ask about any other state or local programs that may be able to provide you with benefits or services.

Now that you have a few more details, do you think that you might be eligible for any of the above state insurance or disability programs? Which ones? Why do you think that you would be eligible? Will you file a claim? Whom will you contact to follow up? Take some time to come up with a plan to get the benefits that you will help you.

Local HIV/AIDS Service Organizations

Before you go searching for HIV/AIDS service organizations and other resources in your area, think a moment about what type of services that you need right now. Do you need counseling, support, medications, food, housing, or health insurance? How about assistance in filing benefit claims or completing legal documents? Put down everything you can think of that would help you right now.

In my experience and travels, I have seen HIV/AIDS service organizations offering everything from medical services to gym memberships to computers. Most of these services are available for free or at a reduced price for people with HIV. Your biggest challenge now is to find these services.

To help guide your search, I have come up with a suggested checklist for you to follow. Number a page in your journal from 1 to 11, and then keep track of your research for each method below that you use. Make notes in your journal during your search so you will be able to follow up your leads later on.

1. Ask your doctor if they know of any these organizations.
2. Contact your local health department.
3. Visit the website of your state's or province's health department.
4. Call your local AIDS Hotline.
5. Check your local phone book for listings using words like *AIDS, HIV,* and *positive.*
6. Ask other HIV-positive people about helpful organizations in your area.
7. Ask people who know your status about any organizations they may know of.
8. Search on the Internet using keywords like *HIV* and *AIDS* in combination with the name of your city or state or province.
9. Check at www.thebody.com for a list of organizations by state and by country.
10. Click on the links button on any HIV- or AIDS-related website that you find.
11. Check for community organizations that serve the general population by providing things like food, housing, and job training.

Hopefully as a result of your search, you have discovered some local organizations that can help you get everything that you need to be okay. It's time now to take advantage of all they have to offer. But before you go, let me ask you this—do you have any fears about using these organizations? Are you afraid of being seen going in and out of their buildings? Are you worried they'll tell other people about your status? Are you concerned that you may be treated poorly or judged somehow? Will this stop you from using their services?

If you could truly benefit from these services, it would be a shame to let your fears stop you from doing so. Try to address them on your own if you can; but if not, definitely consider using a therapist or counselor to help you to move past them and to continue on your journey.

Chapter 4 Checklist

In your journal, number a page from 1 to 19, and then complete the checklist below to mark your progress. Chapter 4 completes your current stage, *Building Your Foundation*. It is imperative that you have a solid foundation under you before you start to consider how HIV affects your daily life. **DO NOT** move on to the next stage in Chapter 5 until you have accomplished every item on the checklists in Chapters 1 through 4.

Federal Programs

1. Identified if you have ever received benefits from any federal programs, if you have paid Social Security tax, or if you have paid retirement tax to another program like PERS

2. Identified if you currently have a disability that prevents you from working and if it is HIV-related

3. Determined if you are likely to get a Social Security Administration (SSA) disability determination, using the SSA's publication and your local HIV/AIDS service organization for guidance

4. Determined if you might be eligible for SSDI, SSI or Medicare benefits, using the SSA or your local HIV/AIDS service organization for guidance

5. Filed claims for benefits from these federal programs if you are eligible, contacting each federal program or your local HIV/AIDS service organization for help in filing

6. Acknowledged that Medicare doesn't start until 24 months after you start receiving SSDI, doesn't cover prescription drugs and isn't valid outside the U.S.

7. Checked with your state or your local HIV/AIDS service organization to see what other benefits you are entitled to receive if you are eligible for SSI benefits

8. Followed up with your local HIV/AIDS service organization to see if there are other federal programs that may benefit you

State Programs

9. Identified if you have ever received Medicaid or state disability benefits before or if you are still receiving them now

10. Determined if you are eligible for Medicaid benefits, knowing you may automatically qualify for them if you are receiving SSI benefits

11. Determined if your state has a short-term disability plan and if you are eligible for benefits

12. Recognized that if you paid tax to a state retirement program like PERS instead of Social Security, you might be eligible for disability benefits from that state program

13. Contacted your local HIV/AIDS service organization for assistance in filing claims and to see if there are other state programs for which you are eligible, including drug coverage and health insurance premium payments

Local HIV/AIDS Service Organizations

14. Identified what type of things and services that you need right now
15. Acknowledged your feelings and fears about going to these organizations and using their services
16. Recognized that you may have to provide a letter from your doctor confirming your HIV before you can access some services
17. Acknowledged that laws prevent these organizations from disclosing your medical information without your authorization
18. Completed the HIV/AIDS service organization search checklist within the chapter
19. Contacted at least one local HIV/AIDS service organization as a result of your search

Resource Examples

Nolo's Guide to Social Security Disability, David A. Morton, nolopress.com

How to Get SSI & Social Security Disability: An Insider's Step by Step Guide, Mike Davis

Pub. No. 05-10020: A Guide to Social Security and SSI Disability Benefits for People with HIV Infection, Social Security Administration

Medicare for the Clueless: The Complete Guide to This Federal Program, Joan Harkins Conklin

Disability Workbook for Social Security Applicants: Managing Your Application for Disability Insurance Benefits, Douglas M. Smith

Social Security Administration, www.ssa.gov
Look for: Information on benefit programs, getting a disability determination and filing benefit claims

Being Alive, www.beingalive.org
Look for: HIV consumer guidebook geared towards San Diego but full of U.S. national resources, including many great websites

The Body Positive, www.thebody.com
Look for: Lists of HIV/AIDS service organizations for the U.S., Canada and the rest of the world

Council of Religious AIDS Networks, www.aidsfaith.org
Look for: Links to each religion's website where you may find services available for your use

Chapter 5

Things to Consider in Daily Life

By now, your crisis period should be completely behind you and your foundation firmly in place. By that I mean you have calmed down from your emotional and mental turmoil, made some important decisions in laying the groundwork for a peaceful future, and adopted habits that support your long-term health. If you are still having a difficult time accepting your diagnosis, are experiencing anger or depression, or find yourself unable to function normally on a day-to-day basis, stop now and go back to the first two stages in this book. To help ensure the success of your transition to living in peace with HIV, you first need to resolve the issues discussed in those two stages. No shortcuts are allowed, as they will do you no good. The items discussed below in this current stage will be of no assistance in your healing process if you haven't put your crisis behind you back in Chapter 1 or built your foundation in Chapters 2 through 4. Go back now and finish your work to avoid becoming overwhelmed or damaging your emotional and physical health.

If you have successfully completed the first two stages, then you are ready to move forward on your journey. Congratulations on your hard fought progress to this point! Believe me when I tell you that you have made it through the toughest part of your journey. Putting a solid foundation under yourself as you have done is crucial for getting to a state of peace with HIV. Your goal is not far off now. The next stage in your journey, *Managing Your Details,* involves giving some consideration, in light of HIV, to certain details and decisions that will likely pop up in your daily life. Let's start in this chapter with the more personal aspects involved.

Impact on Social Life

How HIV affects your social life may vary to some degree by where you live. Those living in rural communities or in more conservative cities may experience more feelings of isolation or fear of stigma than those living in larger, more progressive cities. Bigger metropolitan regions generally have a large, vocal population of people living with HIV and an extensive number of service organizations to assist them. Smaller communities or more conservative towns may have residents that are HIV-positive, but because of fear of stigma or persecution, they are probably fairly invisible to the other residents. Even if HIV/AIDS service organizations exist in these places, people with HIV may underutilize their services for fear of being seen doing so by other residents. Even though the level of HIV/AIDS awareness and education has grown significantly in recent years, I suspect that attitudes towards HIV/AIDS in these areas are changing at a slower rate.

That being said, let's discuss some issues you will probably face regarding your social life. The first one that comes to mind is dating. Back in your crisis period, you probably thought you would never date again. You will. But at first, your confidence may be shaken. Mine definitely was. I felt damaged. It seemed like my status was the other shoe that was waiting to drop with anyone that I met. The only question was when to drop it. The longer that I waited, the stronger that my fear of its impact grew. The worry that the other person would run away when I told them gnawed at my stomach, causing me tremendous stress. Usually I would find some way to drive people away to avoid telling them, or I would just stop dating them without explanation. I found the whole experience to be awkward and awful, so I decided to start meeting people online instead. Online I could put my status in my profile so that people knew it before they even started talking to me. Call it a coping mechanism. It worked on some level, but relying on the online world long term to provide all your social contacts is a risky proposition. You live most of your life in the real world, and that is where you need to learn to live peacefully with HIV. It took me almost four years to figure that one out, but I hope that my example helps you to adjust a lot more quickly.

The question of when to tell someone about your status still remains. My advice is to tell them when you feel that it is the right time and that you are comfortable with it. However, if a fear about telling them is growing within you, I recommend that you tell them as soon as you can work it in. It is more important to preserve your mental health at this point than to worry about their reaction. If they have an issue with HIV, telling them on the second date or the sixth date won't make any difference. You may be thinking that the longer that you wait, the more that they will get to know you and the less that it will matter to them. Nice theory, I agree, but it doesn't usually work that way in practice. The important thing to focus on is being okay with yourself, no matter what their reaction is.

One thing that may help you adjust to dating now is to join a social group for people with HIV. It is a great opportunity to spend time with people that understand firsthand what you have been through. Meeting people that have lived with HIV for 5, 10, maybe 15 years might help you to believe in a long happy future for yourself. Maybe you will strike up some new friendships and possibly even a relationship. At the very least, you will be out circulating again, gaining confidence and experience in socializing with your new status. If there is no social group in your area, you might try using online chat rooms or personal ads to meet other HIV-positive people in your area. Just be careful not to let anyone fill your head with their horror stories since you are making this your own experience with HIV.

On the flip side, I caution you about socializing only with other people that have HIV. I have met many people that only date or have friendships with other HIV-positive people. While I understand how doing this may feel more comfortable for someone, I am not convinced that it is beneficial for one's long-term happiness. To find that peace that you are looking for, you have to grow comfortable dealing with your status in any social situation, including ones involving people who don't have HIV. If you think about it, you don't want people to accept or reject you based upon HIV, so it stands to reason that you might try not to do it either. Besides, when love comes into your life, it usually ignores all the rules you've set down for it. That means it may come to you in the form of a HIV-negative person. If you have done your mental work around this issue, then perhaps you won't be inclined to run from it out of fear and discomfort. Life may hold many great things for you, but you have to be open and ready to receive them. It's worth the effort to be ready.

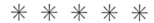

Disclosing Your Status

This seems like a natural topic to follow our discussion about dating. Should you disclose your HIV status to someone you're about to have sex with? If they don't ask, should you tell? Whose responsibility is it? Great questions, as always. For the sake of our discussion now, let's agree that almost every sexual activity that two people do together has some risk of HIV transmission, even if protection is used. This potential risk is the entire reason that disclosing your status is an issue for you to consider. We will talk more about safe sex in the next section.

There are two main trains of thought in use for when to disclose your status. The first, which I operated under for a few years, is very similar to the military policy on gays—if they don't ask, don't tell. The thought is that if the other person doesn't ask about your status, then they don't care if you have HIV. In reality, this isn't always the case. For example, a few years ago I disclosed my status to someone that I was about to be intimate with. He immediately thanked for me for my honesty and said that he never fools around with HIV-positive men. However, I knew that he had slept with a HIV-positive friend of mine, and I also knew that he had never asked my friend about his status. My friend didn't tell. When I confronted this man with what I knew (without telling him my friend's name), he became extremely angry that someone had "deceived" him by not disclosing their status. Clearly, this man cared about having sex with positive people, but he assumed that it was the positive person's responsibility to disclose their status, not his responsibility to ask. My point here is that if you decide to follow this philosophy of not telling unless they ask, make sure that you understand that it doesn't always mean that they don't care. Maybe they just forgot to ask in the heat of the moment. Or perhaps they are thinking it is your duty to tell them. Also, be prepared for the possibility of a backlash down the line if they find out about your status later by some other means. In my case, there was no trouble because I didn't tell this person my friend's name, but it could happen.

The other philosophy about disclosure is one of shared responsibility or full disclosure. In other words, it is your duty to disclose your status as well as the other person's duty to ask you what your status is, and vice versa. With two people taking responsibility for getting the information out there, there is no room for misunderstanding. This way, everyone involved can make an informed choice about what risks that they are taking by being intimate. For me personally, this policy ultimately made the most sense. It allowed me the sense of freedom to completely enjoy my intimate experiences without any feelings or fears of having manipulated or deceived the other person. My goal here is not to be preachy, but rather to point out the benefits and shortfalls of approaches as I have experienced them. By now, I am confident you will take the information I share and use it to make a decision that works for you.

As I mentioned earlier, I know firsthand how difficult and awkward it can be to tell another person face-to-face about your status. Some people have found unique ways to avoid having to say the words. One person I know of had "HIV+" tattooed on his shoulder so that anyone that he was intimate with would see it and know his status. Knowing he couldn't handle the stress of saying the words, he found another way to disclose his status so that the other person would know the risks. Fantastic! I am not advocating that everyone go out and get a tattoo, but you might want to consider other non-verbal methods of disclosing your status if saying the words is too difficult. Maybe you could write it on a card that you hand to the other person. One person that I heard of actually had it printed on a business-style card so he could just hand it out when necessary. You get the idea.

Just as a reminder, in Chapter 2 I discussed that fact that it is a crime in some jurisdictions to knowingly expose another person to HIV without their knowledge. You might want to include this factor in your decision about disclosure.

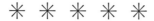

Safe Sex

Some people argue that the only safe sex is the sex that you have by yourself. They point out that any other sexual activity has some risk of disease, making the adjective *safe* inappropriate. Instead of *safe,* they label certain sex acts using protection as *safer.* I understand their point, but for our discussion, it would be more beneficial to focus on the risky behavior itself than how we label it.

There are a variety of opinions about which sexual activities are high or low risk when it comes to transmitting or receiving diseases. I recognize that many of us, myself included, became HIV-positive as a result of sexual activity and might need to reaffirm our idea of safe sex practices. Rather than spending too much time debating differing opinions about what is safe, however, I will leave it to you to consult local HIV/AIDS service organizations or research online for the latest guidance on the risks involved with specific activities since new studies are released all the time. Instead, I would like to focus your attention on a few risky sexual behaviors that I believe merit special consideration.

The first behavior is having unprotected anal or vaginal sex. Even if both people involved already have HIV, there are still significant risks present for both of you. If you are already HIV-positive and then are re-infected with another strain of HIV, your experience with the disease could take a turn for the worse. Some strains are more powerful than others, with more drug resistance. You would probably begin to experience the effects of the stronger strain on your health, possibly running out of treatment options sooner and seeing a decline in your lab results. There is some debate out there about whether more than one strain really exists, but I have seen this happen to people that I have known. Besides HIV, unprotected anal or vaginal sex can expose you to a multitude of other sexually transmitted diseases such as hepatitis, HPV (causes genital and anal warts), syphilis, gonorrhea, herpes, and KSHV (causes Kaposi's Sarcoma, a cancer) just to name a few. There doesn't have to be semen involved for exposure to occur as precum and vaginal fluid have generally been shown to carry the same risk. For every health problem that you add to your body, your long-term health outlook will likely suffer. Without fail, every doctor I have seen has told me that their biggest challenge with HIV is to get their HIV-positive patients to stop having unprotected or unsafe sex. Give some serious consideration as to whether the payoff from this type of activity is worth the immense health risks involved.

The second activity that I want to single out is swallowing semen. I have met people who deem this activity safe because they believe that stomach acid will kill any virus in the semen. I can see what they are thinking logically, but how do they know that this is true? And even if it is true, the semen hits a lot of places on the way down. Any cut or tear in your mouth, gums, throat or stomach is an opening for a virus to be absorbed into your body before your stomach acid could kill it. I can't help but think that this is like swallowing a pill covered with poison, then hoping the poison doesn't get into your system before your stomach acid destroys it. Some people may see this as exciting, but if your goal is to live in peace with HIV, you might want to give some serious consideration to all the risks involved before adopting this sexual behavior.

Finally, some people with HIV believe that if the other person tells you that they don't have HIV, then receiving unprotected anal or vaginal sex from them or swallowing their semen isn't risky behavior. You already know that there are other health risks associated with these behaviors. But even in regard to HIV re-infection, what if this person was lying to you about their status? And even if they were being honest about their status, how does that person truly know that they don't have HIV? They could be infected and not know it yet. Did you know you had HIV at the moment that you became infected? I didn't. The virus could be in an incubation period within that person where it doesn't show up on tests for up to six months or possibly even longer. During this time, the virus can still be transmitted to another person, meaning you. Even if their latest test came back negative, they could have been infected with HIV the next day and not know it. You have no idea what their true status is. The long-standing rule of thumb regarding safe sex is to treat everyone as if they have HIV, for your own protection as well as theirs. Good food for thought in deciding what is safe sex for you.

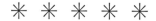

Confidentiality

Your doctor and his or her staff know. Your therapist knows. Some of your family and friends know. Your support network knows. People at the local HIV/AIDS service organization know. That may seem like a lot of people who know your status. What if they all suddenly start telling other people?

As far as the doctor and therapist go, they are legally prevented from disclosing medical information about you without your permission. This legal protection is called doctor-patient confidentiality, and it extends to the doctor's staff as well. If they do make a disclosure of your status without your permission, you will be able to take legal action against them. As I already mentioned in Chapter 2, keep in mind that the law in some jurisdictions may allow or require your doctor to tell your partner and children about your HIV infection.

HIV/AIDS service organizations have well-established confidentiality policies that they usually give to you in writing when you use their services. If they don't give you a copy, ask for one.

The laws that prohibit the disclosure of your medical information without your authorization apply to these organizations as well, so you should be protected. Recent amendments to U.S. federal privacy laws regarding medical information have increased even more this protection for people in the U.S. To protect this privacy, be sure to ask if any forms you sign when enrolling for services are giving the organization permission to disclose your medical information to anyone outside the organization. Some organizations don't identify you by name, using instead an untraceable piece of information like part of your social security number, which may help to ease your fears.

That leaves us with family, friends, past lovers, and people in your support network still to consider. Unfortunately, in most circumstances, there is nothing you can do legally to stop these people from telling others. The laws that stop HIV/AIDS service organizations from disclosing your medical information aren't usually applied to individuals whom you've told on a personal level about your HIV. Your best method for getting them to keep it to themselves may be to flat out ask them not to tell other people. Given that most of these people care about you and your well-being, you can probably rely on them to be discreet. Of course, if they are having a difficult time coping with the news, they may share it with some people in their support network. You may have to trust them to tell these other people to keep your confidence as well. My advice is to tell the people in your life whom you need to tell, ask them to keep it private, and then just go on trust and faith.

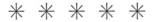

Treatment Management

Your HIV treatment is yours to manage. At this point, it may not seem like you have much control over your treatment, but you really do. I am certain that the story I'm about to tell you will raise some eyebrows in the HIV medical community as well as within some HIV/AIDS service organizations. However, I think my experience will illustrate to you what I mean when I tell you that your treatment really is within your control.

When I first was diagnosed, I went on medications almost right way. My doctor thought it would be the best thing for me to do, and for my peace of mind, I was all for it. For the first two years, everything went well as I just took my drugs and never questioned anything. Then I started to develop the side effect of lipodystrophy, a redistribution of fat away from the limbs and towards the abdomen. I became depressed about the changes in my appearance, so my doctor changed two of my medications to try and stop this problem. Unfortunately, one of the new medications made me feel somewhat dizzy and unfocused at times. My doctor told me I would have to either adjust to the new side effects or go back on the old drugs. I accepted what she said and took the new drugs. The lipodystrophy continued to worsen. As I approached the three-year mark of taking medications, something in my heart told me I should take a break from this treatment. I asked my doctor if I could stop. She said no, that once someone started using HIV medications, they could never completely stop without serious risks. I consulted two other HIV specialists, and both told me the same thing. Stopping was not an option. Period. It didn't matter that my health over the past three years had been very good. The answer was no.

What they were saying just didn't make sense to me intuitively. Protocols for starting people on the medications had changed so much that if I had been diagnosed that day instead of three years ago, they would never have started me on the drugs. I felt trapped into a lifetime of pill popping, side effects, and God knows what. So I decided that I had to do what my heart told me to do—take a leap of faith and stop the medications.

When I told my current doctor that I was going to stop medications, she told me that if I did so, I faced the risk of the virus mutating to where it would become resistant to one or more drugs, reducing my treatment options. I asked her if she could tell me the long-term risks of taking the drugs, and she said that nobody really knows yet because the drugs are still too new. I decided to face the risk I knew rather than the one

I didn't. It was my own choice, my own treatment, and my own life. I decided if stopping didn't work out, I could start the medications again with the understanding that they might not work as well. I made my choice knowing all the potential risks and benefits and was prepared to accept both.

The reason for telling you this story is not to advocate that you stop taking your drugs. On the contrary, if the drugs are helping you and you feel okay about taking them, then it sounds like you are doing what works for you. Rather, the point of my story is to illustrate that you are in complete control of what treatment that you get for HIV. You are free to seek out and accept or deny any treatment that you desire. You and you alone experience the benefits and consequences of your treatment choices. Don't let any doctor convince you that pills are your only option, be it for HIV or any other condition. An old saying states that there are always three options in every circumstance, even if none is very appealing. Remember this—while your doctor or other professionals you encounter during your treatment for HIV may be concerned about your health, you are the only one concerned with managing your life. In other words, the only way you are ever going to live in peace with HIV is to cause it to happen for yourself. Your life, your choices.

So after my story, you're probably wondering how things have turned out for me. So far, so good. After two years off medications, my health and my lab results have both been better than I expected. Even my doctor was surprised at my lab results at first, asking me a few times if I really had stopped taking my medications. But let me make something crystal clear— I didn't just stop my medications and pray. I made significant changes to my life first before stopping. Luckily, I already didn't smoke, drink, take drugs, or consume caffeine. But I knew that for me to live in peace with HIV, I would also have to focus on healing my mind, body, and spirit as they are all tied together in determining my well-being. I started eating an organic, nutritionally balanced diet, adopted a disciplined workout program, and began meditating and doing yoga. I started consuming a multitude of supplements, including herbal treatments, and dedicating myself to getting at least eight hours of sleep each night. In addition, I left my stressful job environment, began exploring my faith and spirituality, and enlisted the help of a therapist and some holistic practitioners. In other words, I did everything I could to put a healthy foundation under my choice, and so far it has been working beautifully. The way I was living before wasn't doing anything to support my long-term health or my goal of living in peace with HIV. Now I have a renewed vigor for life, am at peace with HIV, and am ready and eager to help you make the same journey towards peace. My hope is that someday this will be your story too, regardless of what treatment options you choose.

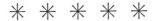

Discrimination

You told your boss that you have HIV, and then you are passed over for a promotion. The desk clerk at a hotel tells you that there were no rooms available, yet you notice that there are barely any cars in the parking lot and it is already 10:00 p.m. Have you been discriminated against because you have HIV? Maybe. Maybe not. That is the problem with proving discrimination. It is in the minds of the people discriminating, and short of developing telepathic skills to read their minds, you can't be sure what is motivating their actions unless they make some blatant or obvious comments. Since the fact that you have HIV is not often apparent by looking at you, it can't be assumed that someone knew about your status at the time of their action unless you can prove that they did.

In the U.S., the federal Americans with Disabilities Act (ADA) prohibits discrimination against persons with disabilities, which includes HIV/AIDS. The biggest area of application of this law so far has been in the employment area, where employers are required to make reasonable accommodations for your disability so that you can continue to work. The ADA also specifically prohibits discrimination in places of public accommodation, meaning locations like restaurants, hotels, airports, and sports arenas. Unfortunately, not many cases have ever been decided under the ADA to give us clear guidance as to what is considered discrimination. Most cases are settled out of court mainly because companies don't want to be the one that tests the ADA in court and loses in a big way.

So why am I telling you this? Because I want you to know that discrimination protection does exist for you out there, at least in theory. But really, my main goal here is for you to be careful not to let the worry of being discriminated against be your undoing. If you adopt the mindset that having HIV is the cause of every denial, failure, or missed opportunity that occurs in your life, you may find that the fear of discrimination has become more disabling than HIV may ever be. If, however, you do strongly suspect that you have been discriminated against because of your status, contact your local HIV/AIDS service organization for legal assistance or consult an attorney directly. Just remember that to live in peace with HIV, you will need to achieve a realistic perspective of how having HIV plays into the events of your daily life.

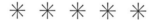

Freedom to Travel

Now that you know that you have HIV, you might be thinking that your traveling days are over. You may feel that you need to stay close to home in case you become ill and require medical attention. And international travel may seem completely out of the question because of the chance that you could get sick from something you eat or drink while you are far from home.

Actually, you still have more freedom than you might think. If you are traveling within the U.S. and have health insurance, then you are probably covered for any emergency medical treatment you might need on the road. Some plans also provide coverage for routine illnesses while you are out of town, though usually at much lower coverage rates. Unless you currently have a serious HIV-related illness, any competent doctor should be able to treat a routine illness that pops up while you are away from home. How colds and the flu affect you now shouldn't be much different than before you had HIV, unless your immune system has been weakened immensely over time. At the time I was diagnosed, I was traveling 75% of the time, all over the country. I experienced quite a few colds and bouts with flu while away from home, but nothing unusual happened. Of course, a serious illness or injury could strike anyone anywhere, resulting in the need for emergency treatment. If this happens to you, ask the person treating you to have your doctor consult by phone if that would make you more comfortable. You might consider telling the treating person about your status, to ensure they fully understand your medical condition. While I was traveling, I was lucky enough to have a doctor who would let me call her directly if any illness surfaced, and that took a load off my mind.

For international trips, it is sometimes difficult to avoid getting sick from something you eat or drink. Your likelihood of illness may be less in more developed countries than in third world nations, but it still exists anywhere. The same general travel tips you're probably already aware of still apply: drink only bottled water, don't get ice in your drinks, and only eat food that appears fresh and is from a sanitary restaurant. Buying anything to eat from street vendors in most foreign countries is taking a pretty big risk of ending up sick. One extra tip is to only drink bottled water on airplanes, not water from the plane's tanks, as studies have shown these tanks to be packed with bacteria. Skip ice on planes for the same reason, as well as tea or coffee made with water from the tanks. If you aren't certain whether tank water was used in making your beverage, then just ask.

If you do happen to get sick while out of the country, don't panic. These types of illnesses can be uncomfortable but are rarely life threatening. In the past four years, I have been to countries on almost every continent for work and for fun, and I have guzzled my share of Pepto-Bismol® to stop stomach upset and diarrhea. It usually only lasts a few days. If your illness continues for more than a week, however, or gets increasingly severe, you might need to use antibiotics to kill the offending bacteria in your system. Have your doctor prescribe an antibiotic to take with you just in case, but use it only if the condition persists or worsens. You don't want to put any drugs in your body unless you need them, and overuse of antibiotics can lead to resistance to their effects in the future when you might truly need them. As always, for serious illness or injury, get medical attention right away and worry about insurance or costs afterwards. Protecting your life is your first priority. Here again, you may want to tell anyone treating you about your status so that they fully understand your medical condition.

Legally, you should be aware that a few countries have laws allowing them to deny entry to visitors with HIV. You might be surprised to find out that the U.S., Canada, and the United Kingdom are among them. Thankfully, however, this legal restriction appears to be rarely enforced in these three countries. Personally, I have traveled back and forth between all three countries several times without incident. Most countries do require an AIDS test for foreigners staying more than 90 days or who are applying for residency or a work permit. Regardless of which country you live in, check the U.S. Department of State website for more information on current entry restrictions for countries around the world. It is also a good idea to contact the closest embassy of the country you want to visit to find out their latest policy. You might be able to find out that same information on their website. Consult your local HIV/AIDS service organization for assistance if you are having difficulty finding the information that you need.

So how would anyone know that you have HIV when you are trying to enter a country? I guess they could ask you directly, though I have never heard or read of this happening. One thing I have heard is that some customs officials are trained to recognize the name of HIV medications, so your pill bottle may give you away if you happen to have your bags searched. Rather than leave the pills at home and risk their health, some people I know have put their pills in unmarked plastic bags. To give you some perspective on this topic, I know a scientist who has traveled to hundreds of countries in the past six years, carrying his HIV medications in their bottles and never once having a hassle, despite the occasional luggage search. You would probably have a better chance of winning the lottery than getting turned away at the border for having HIV, but you should know that it is possible in some parts of the world. If by some twist of fate this does happen to you, at least you can feel good about putting your health first as you take the long plane ride back home.

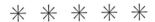

Helpful Exercises

Let's start this new stage by focusing on how HIV might play a part in your daily life. How do you think it will come up in day-to-day activities? What areas in your life seem the most likely to be affected by HIV? What feelings and fears do you have about dealing with HIV in these areas? What are you afraid will happen now that you have HIV?

Remember to reread often what you have written here as you work through the following exercises. It is important for you to consider your feelings and fears if your goal is to draft a plan of action that fits your life for each topic below.

Impact on Social Life

After you heard your diagnosis, one of your first thoughts might have been about how this was going to affect your social life, including dating. How do you think HIV will affect your social life? How will it affect dating and making new friends? What are your feelings and fears surrounding this? What do you think might happen when you try to meet new people?

Let's start your work in this area with dating. You might have felt like damaged goods after you found out you had HIV, maybe thinking that you would never date again. You will, I promise. Perhaps you already have. If you have had a date since your diagnosis, how did it go? Did you feel comfortable or uneasy? Did this person already know your status? If not, did you tell them at any point before, during or after the date? What happened? What are your fears about telling your status to someone that you are interested in? Capture all the details in your journal.

Now that you know where your mind stands on this topic, let's talk a bit more about meeting people to date. How do you meet them now after your diagnosis? Do you meet them in bars, online, or maybe through friends? Have you decided not to try and meet people? What are your fears about meeting people? Have you met or dated any HIV-positive people? Are you afraid HIV-negative people that you meet might reject you? There are lots of questions here that need your answers.

So now you know what is stopping you from getting back out there and meeting people to date. To find your peace with HIV, however, you must find a way to deal with your fears and become comfortable again in these types of social situations. Can you get past these issues on your own? Will time help you, or do you think that maybe using a counselor or therapist may be a better solution? What ideas do you have for making this transition?

Of course, most new people that we meet become friends instead of dates. Have you thought about how you might make some new friends? Are you worried that they might reject you as a friend if they found out about your status? If you don't already have friends who have HIV, are you interested in making some? What would be the benefits and drawbacks of making some HIV-positive friends? What are your fears in this area?

Take a moment to begin drafting a plan for how you will handle your social life now that you have HIV. Be sure to include any changes you will make to your current methods for meeting people, any new methods you will use to meet them, and any methods you will definitely avoid. Consider how you will meet both HIV-negative and HIV-positive people for friendship or dating. Having a plan may help to keep you from becoming isolated and detached, conditions that will likely stall your progress on your journey.

Disclosing Your Status

Disclosing your status in this context refers to telling your status to someone with whom you're about to be sexually intimate. What are your feelings and fears about telling someone your status in this situation? Would you tell them before you had sex if they asked? How about if they didn't ask? Would you tell them if during sex they wanted to do something that you thought might put them at risk of getting HIV from you?

As a reminder, there are two main approaches to disclosure out there. The first is don't ask, don't tell. If they don't ask you about your status, then you don't tell them because it must not matter to them. The second approach is one of full disclosure. This requires you both to disclosure your status and ask the other person about theirs. What is your feeling on the duty to disclose? What seems like the right approach for you? Why? Do you have any fears about using it? Do you think it would be too difficult for you to say the words? Are you concerned with being rejected or having the other person react violently?

If you answered the two sets of questions above, then you have all the information you need to form a strategy for this topic. Disclosure is such a personal decision. Only you only can understand which approach will best fit your life. Use your journal to design an approach you would feel comfortable using. Consider what you would say to the other person, when you would say it, and what non-verbal method, if any, you would use to get the point across if necessary. A little planning now could save you from many awkward and emotional moments in the future.

Safe Sex

Safe sex or safer sex? Rather than getting hung up on which label to use, let's discuss what it means to you. How do you define safe sex? What activities do you deem safe and unsafe? What is your basis for this?

The concept of what is safe sex is open to some debate. Medical studies come out all the time adding to our knowledge and possibly confusion about which activity is safe and which is not. Using your definition of safe sex from the above question, do you currently have safe sex? If you do, what things are you doing that makes it safe? If you don't, what things have you done that may not be safe? Be honest for your own benefit. Nobody is going to use what you write here to judge you.

Below is a current list of some sex practices generally considered to be safe or unsafe. Keep in mind that this list is subjective and open to interpretation. I encourage you to do more research and decide on your own which practices are safe or not. There are safe sex guidelines all over the Internet at websites like the Center for Disease Control, www.cdc.gov/hiv and The Body Positive, www.thebody.com. But for our discussion here today, this list is sufficient. It is broken down into *safe* meaning no risk, *safer* meaning some risk, and *unsafe* meaning really big risk.

Sexual Practice	Category
Masturbation, Non-sexual Massage, Abstinence	Safe
Hand Jobs (no fluid)	Safe
Oral Sex with Condom	Safer
Vaginal or Anal Sex with Condom	Safer
Hand Job with Condom (fluid)	Safer
Oral Sex without Condom	Safer/Unsafe
Vaginal or Anal Sex without Condom	Unsafe
Swallowing Semen or Vaginal Fluid	Unsafe

Keep in mind that the greatest risk occurs when blood or sexual fluid touches the soft, moist inside areas of the mouth, nose, rectum, vagina, or tip of the penis. Knowing what you now know, go back and evaluate your last answer about your sex practices. How does it match up to the list? Are you having safe sex? Are there things you did that you thought were safe but now might not be? What are they?

In our discussion of safe sex, you have probably been thinking mostly about HIV infection as the risk involved. However, remember that the list of other sexually transmitted diseases (STDs) that you can catch from unsafe sex is quite long. If a sexual partner tells you that they don't have HIV or other

STDs, do you follow the same safe sex guidelines as before or use different practices? Do you take more risks with your own health in these situations? If the other person has HIV, do you still follow the safe sex guidelines or use different practices? Do you take more risks with your own health in these situations?

Hopefully you have done a lot of thinking and learning while completing the exercises in this topic. Has your notion of safe sex changed now? Have you decided to make any changes to your behavior? Take a few moments now to come up with your safe sex plan in your journal, including what you think is safe and unsafe behavior. Protecting your health and your future is worth the time.

Confidentiality

During your crisis period, you probably told a lot of people about your status. This might have included your doctor, therapist, family, friends, partner, and people at your local HIV/AIDS service organization. What are your feelings and fears about confidentiality? Whom do you think might tell other people about your status? Whom are you worried will find out about your HIV? How do you think they will find out? What will happen if they do?

Non-disclosure laws prevent doctors, therapists, and anyone else that treats you for HIV from disclosing your status without your permission. Unfortunately, these non-disclosure laws don't normally apply to people whom you've told on a personal level about your status. Hopefully, you took their trustworthiness and caring for you into consideration before you told them. Is there anyone you forgot to tell to keep it private? Is there someone you told that you are worried about telling others? Do you need to reconfirm your wishes to these people? Make some notes in your journal and create a plan for you to tie up your loose ends regarding confidentiality. It may help to ease your mind.

Treatment Management

Even though it may not seem like it at times, your treatment for HIV is yours to manage. It is completely within your control. Because of this, your relationship with your doctor is very important. How active are you in deciding your treatment? How interactive is your relationship with your doctor? Do you accept everything your doctor says? Are you comfortable doing that? Do you ask questions? Have you ever obtained a second opinion regarding a recommendation that your doctor made?

If you are on HIV medications, which ones are you taking? What side effects have you experienced, if any? How did you deal with them? What did the doctor say or recommend that you do when you told him or her about the side effects? Were you comfortable with your doctor's comments or recommendations? Did you do any outside research?

My goal is to have you recognize the degree to which you are managing your treatment for HIV. To find your peace with HIV, you must adopt an approach with which you are truly comfortable. If, for example, you want to question your doctor's decisions but you never do, then you haven't found an approach that you can live peacefully with.

Now that you understand better how you have been managing your treatment, are there any changes that you want to make? Would you like to be more or less aggressive in your relationship with your doctor, or are things just fine the way they are? Do you feel in comfortable control of your treatment? Have you tried to make changes in the past but didn't because of strong resistance from your doctor? Why did you let it drop? Take some time now to write down what your feelings and desires are for managing your HIV treatment. It is all for you to create and control.

Discrimination

Has fear of being discriminated against because of your HIV entered your mind? What do you think this type of discrimination is? What form does it take? What type of events do you imagine when you think of this type of discrimination? In what types of places do you imagine this discrimination occurring?

The most difficult part of claiming discrimination of any type is proving it actually occurred. Do you think you've been discriminated against because you have HIV? If not, imagine for a moment that you do think that. How could you prove that you having HIV motivated the other person's action? How would the other person know that you have HIV? Can you prove that they knew your status when they took that action?

Without reading someone's mind, it may be difficult to prove that they acted the way they did because of your HIV status, unless they say or write something that is outright discriminatory. Unless that actually did happen, at this point you should probably be more concerned with your own behavior.

Are you seeing discrimination everywhere in your life? Every time someone denies you something, gives you a weird look, or acts rudely towards you, does the thought cross your mind that it's because of your HIV? Be honest with yourself as you try to remember if you have had these feelings. Take a moment to record any of them in your journal.

If left unchecked, your fear of being discriminated against may become more disabling than HIV might ever be for you. Most people have no way of knowing you have HIV, so don't go looking for problems that are likely not there. Do what you can to drop your fears and keep moving forward on this healthy path you are on.

Existing anti-discrimination laws in the U.S. focus mainly on requiring employers to give disabled employees reasonable accommodations in the workplace, within limits. Do you think you need an accommodation at work because of a disabling condition associated with HIV/AIDS? Another type of disability? What changes in your job or workspace need to be made for you to continue working at your company? Have you already made such a request? If so, what happened?

My best advice regarding discrimination is to know your rights and protections, and then just get out there and live your life in the way you always have. If you are finding that a difficult thing to do, then consider getting some counseling to assist you.

Freedom to Travel

Do you feel like you can't go far from home now that you have HIV? What feelings and fears do you have about traveling? Are you afraid that you will get sick or be discriminated against? Are you afraid that you won't get the medical attention that you need?

You've probably traveled to places in your country in the past, and perhaps to other countries as well. Have you ever gotten sick while away from home? What happened? What did you do to treat it? Did you need to seek medical attention? Did you have any fears about being sick while away from home?

Remember, unless you already have a serious HIV-related illness or an extremely weak immune system, routine illnesses probably won't affect you any differently than they did in the past. No matter where you are, you should be able to get effective medical treatment, if necessary.

Before you jet off to your next destination, take some time now in your journal to come up with a plan to give yourself some extra peace of mind when on the road. Determine how you will deal with routine illnesses as you travel. Research what your health insurance will cover when you are away from home, both in your own country and abroad. Perhaps you can even set up an arrangement with your doctor that he or she will be available for you to call for health advice in these situations. Your good health is priority number one and well worth investing this time and effort now.

Chapter 5 Checklist

Before you continue on to Chapter 6, number a page in your journal from 1 to 43, and then complete the checklist below. Managing how HIV affects your daily life is an important part of living in peace with HIV each day. You should finish all the items in this checklist before you move to the next stage in Chapter 7.

First Step:

1. Acknowledged how you think HIV will affect areas of your daily life and what fears and feelings you have about these effects

Impact on Social Life

2. Acknowledged how you think HIV will affect your social life and what feelings and fears you have about these effects

3. Determined how you would handle telling someone that you are dating about your HIV, including when you would tell them or if you would tell them at all

4. Acknowledged your fears and feelings about meeting people to date and what methods you are using to meet people now that you have HIV

5. Considered if you are interested in making friends with more people who have HIV, how you will meet them, and if you have any fears about doing so

6. Remembered not to internalize other people's stories about HIV as your own, once you start meeting other HIV-positive people

7. Considered the fact that having only people with HIV for dates and friends may hinder you in learning to be comfortable in social situations that include both HIV-negative and HIV-positive people

8. Designed and began following a plan to meet people for friendship or dating, now that you have HIV

Disclosing Your Status

9. Acknowledged your feelings and fears about disclosing your status to someone that you are about to be sexually intimate with

10. Evaluated the two main disclosure approaches and determined which one, if either, works for you

11. Acknowledged it may be a crime in your jurisdiction to knowingly expose someone to HIV without their knowledge
12. Devised a non-verbal method to disclosure your status to someone if you find saying the words too difficult

Safe Sex

13. Determined what you think is safe sex, including which activities you consider safe or unsafe
14. Acknowledged if you currently have safe sex or not, and what things you are doing or not doing to make it safe or unsafe
15. Researched and acknowledged what current safe sex guidelines are
16. Reevaluated your sexual practices against your research and determined if some things you thought were safe are not
17. Acknowledged that unsafe sex exposes you to other illnesses like herpes, hepatitis and syphilis as well as re-infection with a more power strain of HIV
18. Determined if you follow different safe sex practices with HIV-negative or HIV-positive people
19. Accepted that the other person might be lying about being HIV-negative or not yet know they have been infected with HIV
20. Used what you learned in the chapter to create and begin to follow a safe sex plan to protect your health and your future

Confidentiality

21. Acknowledged your feelings and fears about your HIV status being kept confidential
22. Recognized that confidentiality laws prevent doctors and organizations from disclosing your medical information without your permission
23. Accepted that these laws don't normally apply to people whom you've told on a personal level

24. Remembered to ask the people you've told to keep your status private
25. Created and followed a plan to tie up your loose ends about confidentiality, including possibly reminding some people to keep your status private

Treatment Management

26. Identified how interactive your relationship with your doctor currently is and how you feel about this level of interaction
27. Identified what HIV medications, if any, you are taking, their side effects, and how your doctor has dealt with those side effects
28. Accepted that you are in control of your medical treatment for HIV, no matter what other people may tell you
29. Recognized that regardless of whether you let the doctor call all the shots, question the doctor's recommendations or aggressively manage your medical treatment, you need to be completely comfortable with the style of treatment management you have chosen to follow
30. Identified changes, if any, you would like to make to your treatment management style
31. Created and began to follow a plan to achieve the treatment management style you would like to have

Discrimination

32. Identified if you think you've been discriminated against because of HIV and how you know that your HIV was the reason for that person's action
33. Researched and acknowledged the laws that protect you from discrimination because of HIV and what type of actions may be discriminatory
34. Identified if you have an HIV-related or other disability that requires an accommodation by your employer

in order for you to keep working, and filed a request if appropriate

35. Accepted that you can't let the fear of discrimination because of HIV become disabling or prevent you from living your life
36. Determined if you have actually been discriminated against because of your HIV
37. Contacted your local HIV/AIDS service organization for information on discrimination laws and assistance in filing any discrimination claims

Freedom to Travel

38. Acknowledged your feelings and fears about traveling now that you have HIV
39. Acknowledged that you may have been sick in the past while away from home, both in your country and abroad
40. Realized that unless you have a serious HIV-related illness or weak immune system, routine illnesses probably won't affect you any differently than in the past
41. Asked your doctor what you can do to take care of routine or emergency illnesses while away from home
42. Checked with your health insurance company or government health service about your coverage while traveling in your country and abroad
43. Researched the entry requirements regarding HIV for countries that you plan to visit short or long term

Resource Examples

The Guide to Living with HIV Infection, John G. Bartlett

Living Well with HIV and AIDS, Allen Gifford

What if Everything You Thought You Knew about AIDS was Wrong?, Christine Maggliore

Love in The Time of HIV: The Gay Man's Guide To Sex, Dating and Relationships, Michael Mancilla and Lisa Troshinsky

National AIDS Manual Glossary, NAM Publications, www.nam.org.uk

Your Rights in the Workplace, Barbara Kate Repa

HIV/AIDS: Practical, Medical, and Spiritual Guidelines for Daily Living When You're HIV-Positive, Mark Jenkins and Robert E. Larsen

Chinese Medicine for Maximum Immunity, Jason Elias, et al

New York Times Guide to Alternative Health, Jane E. Brody, et al

Alive and Well, www.aliveandwell.org
Look for: Alternative view of how HIV works and what treatments are necessary

Project Inform, www.projinf.org
Look for: Guidance on developing interactive doctor-patient relationship for better treatment

Love in The Time of HIV, www.hivandrelationships.com
Look for: Helpful guidance on disclosure and safe sex issues

AmFar, www.amfar.org
Look for: Latest information about clinical drug trials, treatment protocols and research efforts

U.S. Department of State, travel.state.gov
Look for: Travel publications that list the latest HIV/AIDS entry restrictions by country

Dr. Lark Lands, www.larrylands.com/lark
Look for: Guidance on disease management including use of supplements

AIDS Research Information Center,
www.criticalpath.org/aric/
Look for: PWA/AIDS links that lead to listing of alternative and complementary therapies

The Body Positive, www.thebody.com
Look for: Articles about disclosing your status socially or at work, and safe sex practices

AIDS Education Global Information System, www.aegis.com
Look for: Information about treatment approaches and discrimination laws

The New Mexico AID InfoNet, www.aidsinfonet.org
Look for: Listing of more than 500 AIDS-related websites, broken down by category

Avert.Org, www.avert.org
Look for: Global HIV/AIDS information, including special sections for the UK and Africa

Chapter 6

Addressing Financial and Legal Concerns

Since your diagnosis, I am certain you've had at least a few thoughts about money. Maybe you were wondering how you would support yourself if you became ill. Or maybe you were trying to decide if you should spend all your retirement savings now or keep socking money away as you did before. Back in your crisis state, when your death probably seemed right around the corner, you may have thought about who should get your favorite personal possessions, or who would be the best person to pull the plug if you ended up on life support. Even though your mind wasn't ready to realistically deal with those things, you were on the right track as far as decisions you might consider making about your financial and legal affairs.

The decisions to consider in these areas are basically the same ones you faced before you were diagnosed, but having HIV now does put a little different spin on most of them for you. As part of your current stage, let's review some of these financial and legal decisions in more detail. If you live outside of the U.S., you may need to do some research on how each topic below is handled within your country. Hopefully, the general discussion under each topic and the corresponding exercises will still be beneficial to you as you work through these areas.

Insurance

Health, life, and disability insurance policies become even more valuable assets for people with HIV. These types of insurance protect your financial resources, get you access to affordable quality health care, and ensure that your loved ones are financially secure in the case of your death. If you don't already have these types of insurance, however, you will have a difficult time getting them on your own now. Let me tell you why.

By U.S. insurance industry standards, if you have HIV, you are generally considered uninsurable for these types of policies. This means that if you apply for an individual health, life, or disability insurance policy, you will almost definitely be denied. The reason is that from a business standpoint, your policy would almost certainly be a money loser for these companies as your claims related to your HIV will likely far exceed the insurance premiums that you pay. It is simple math. And I guarantee you that every insurer will ask you about any past or present illnesses or symptoms, so there is no legal way to avoid telling them about your HIV. Leaving it off your application opens you up to being prosecuted for fraud, and that kind of stress is the last thing that you need in your life.

But how can they find out that you have HIV if you don't tell them? I posed that very question to an insurance fraud examiner I know. He told me that the minute that you file any type of claim related to HIV, the insurance company is going to review your application again to see if you disclosed having HIV. After that, they will request your medical records to see if you had been treated for HIV in the past. Every insurance application you sign contains language that allows them to get your medical records. Once they have proof that you lied, you will likely lose your insurance, have to reimburse them for any claims paid on your behalf, and be prosecuted to the fullest extent of the law. He said that his company rarely loses these types of cases. So I guess the message is to think long and hard before you omit HIV or any other illness from an insurance application, and be ready to accept the potential ramifications if you do.

However, your hope of being insured is not lost. You can usually get these types of insurance through your employer if your position includes benefits. The reason is that employer plans are group policies that don't require any proof of insurability. Just by virtue of being an employee of your company, you are eligible to be covered, no questions asked. Just be certain to enroll in these plans when they are first offered to you, because if you decline them and then change your mind later, the insurance company sometimes requires proof of insurability to add you to the group policy. Of course, having HIV now, you will never be able to give them this. That is just the way most insurance contracts with employers are written, unfortunately. Another type of insurance that some employers offer their employees is long-term care plans, which pay for you to reside in a nursing home or other type of custodial facility or to receive home health care. This might be a good insurance for you to choose for added protection in the future.

If you are fortunate, your employer offers more than one health insurance option to their employees. Should you change options now that you have HIV? Let me answer that by sharing my own story. I was in an HMO offered through my employer at the time that I was diagnosed. Shortly thereafter, my employer held an annual open enrollment period where employees could choose to move between different health insurance options. In addition to the HMO, my company offered a more traditional insurance option that allowed me to go to any doctor in or out of their network and still be covered to some degree. In exchange for this freedom, the company charged higher premiums, deductibles and co-pays for this option. I was convinced that I needed that kind of freedom that my HMO didn't offer, just in case I got terribly sick. I switched plans and prepared to pay an extra $1,400 a year in premiums. My current doctor took both insurance plans, so I got to keep her in the bargain. Well, a year went by and nothing unusual happened with my health. When open enrollment came around again, I switched back to the HMO to save money.

What I learned from this whole expensive experience was that it was my doctor and her approach to my treatment that really mattered, not my insurance. That is not to say that some plans haven't denied people the appropriate care that they needed. Our legal system has seen plenty of those cases. But for routine care and established procedures, whether you have a more restrictive plan or one with more freedom might not make that much of a difference as long as you have a good physician guiding your treatment. When deciding what is right for you, weigh the costs against the risk of not getting the services you might need someday, and then choose the option that gives you the most peace of mind.

Let's say something happens and you leave your job. Is all your insurance lost? Whether you lose your life and disability insurance provided through your employer depends upon the terms of the plan. Some plans allow you to convert your policy into an individual policy without providing proof of insurability or allow you to continue to participate in your employer's plan if you pay the full premiums yourself. Check with your employer's plan administrator to see if you have these options.

If your employer has 20 or more employees, then the federal law COBRA gives you the option to keep your same health insurance coverage for up to 18 months if you pay the full premium to your now former employer. You may be eligible for up to 29 months if you received a SSA disability determination within 60 days of leaving your job. You may also be eligible for COBRA if you keep your job but lose your health insurance for some reason, like cutting back to part-time hours.

Keep in mind that with COBRA, you have to pay the full monthly cost of your health insurance to your former employer, even if they weren't passing that cost on to you in the form of a monthly premium. Be prepared for a shock, though, as this premium may be $300 a month or more just for you, and twice that if you have family coverage. After COBRA coverage expires, the federal law HIPAA requires that you be offered an individual insurance policy without having to provide proof of insurability. These federal extensions can be lifesavers. Just don't miss a premium payment on any of this extended coverage or you will most likely get your insurance permanently cut off in a hurry. I saw this happen time and time again when I worked at the federal agency that handles these types of complaints. Usually there was nothing that we could do to get the insurance back for the person involved. If you are having problems making your health insurance premium payments, check with your local HIV/AIDS service organization to see if your state has a program where they will pay your premium for you.

If you do find yourself without health insurance, there are federal and state health insurance programs that you may qualify for including the ones that I discussed in Chapter 4. Contact your local HIV/AIDS service organization for more information and assistance in applying.

✳ ✳ ✳ ✳ ✳

Rainy Day Savings

I don't know how many times in my life I have heard or read the advice that you should have three to six months of living expenses in the bank in case you are out of work. Usually I just roll my eyes and say, yeah, that is a nice dream, but if I had that kind of money lying around, working wouldn't be an issue! My birth certificate doesn't say Rockefeller on it, darn it. But all kidding aside, the underlying message of the advice seems to be a good one.

Life throws us a curve every now and then, and sometimes having enough financial resources to help you through one of those times will reduce the amount of stress involved. If you don't have a savings account or some other easily accessible investment account, then give consideration to starting one. If you can't afford to do that, however, don't stress about it. But even just a few bucks a week dropped into an account or stashed in a secret place might add up to some great peace of mind.

When choosing where to put this money, you might want to stay away from anything that locks up your savings for long periods of time like certain CDs. Also, unless you have the stomach for it, I would suggest that you avoid investing your rainy day funds in volatile investments like stock, the value of which might rise or drop very rapidly in just one day. The point of putting this particular money away is to have it available as soon as you need it, so try to keep that goal in mind if you decide to create a rainy day fund for yourself and your peace of mind.

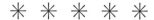

Retirement Planning

I bet that for a while there, the concept of actually reaching retirement age seemed unrealistic to you. You may have considered having a good time now by spending your retirement savings since you weren't going to live very long. Maybe you have already done it. Whatever the situation, I hope that by being present focused and making HIV your own experience, you have been able to stop your mind from convincing you that a long-term future is out of the question. The reality is you may live to be 100 or instead get run over by a bus tomorrow. That doesn't make you any different from everyone else in the world. Many people will live way past retirement age, and others will die far short of it. You are no exception. If you decide not to continue planning for the future, you may well end up there anyway with far too few resources to support your long-term needs.

You might be concerned about locking your money into your company's retirement plan instead of putting it into a savings account where it is readily available for emergencies. However, these retirement funds may be more accessible than you think. Many retirement plans, like the 401(k) plan, allow you to borrow from your account if you need money for emergencies. They charge interest for these loans, but since you are borrowing from yourself, all the interest actually goes back to your account. Interesting, huh? Loan payments are usually deducted from your regular paychecks until the loan is paid off. Also, if you prefer to avoid a loan and make a flat out withdrawal of funds from your 401(k) account, some plans allow for a hardship withdrawal if you meet certain criteria. These withdrawals are usually subject to income tax since 401(k) contributions are not normally taxed when you put them into your account. In addition, the IRS will levy a penalty of 10% on

401(k) withdrawals made before you are age 59 1/2. This penalty can be waived for a few reasons, such as withdrawing funds to pay medical bills. These taxes and penalties also apply to most IRA's and other similar retirement accounts. Definitely check with plan representatives or your financial advisor before taking any loans or withdrawals to ensure you have considered all the options in making your decision.

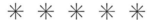

Power of Attorney

You have no doubt heard of a power of attorney but might not know exactly what it is. A power of attorney is a legal form on which you give someone the power to make financial and legal decisions on your behalf, excluding health care decisions. You determine how much power to give this person, how long they have it, and under what circumstances they are able to exercise it. Once you complete this document, you give a copy to the person to whom you granted the power so they can present the document as necessary to carry out your business.

In the context of HIV, it is generally used to designate someone to take over your business affairs if you become incapacitated or otherwise unable to make decisions. Once you regain your decision-making capacity, the current power of attorney period ends and the designated person can no longer exercise the powers you gave them. However, the document still remains valid for any future period of incapacity that meets its terms. In other words, you only need to execute it once to for it to be in effect for any incapacity or series of incapacities you might experience. You will need to review it from time to time, however, to make sure that it still meets your needs and reflects what you feel comfortable with, especially if you haven't included an expiration date within the document. Otherwise, someone you might no longer trust but forgot to remove from the power of attorney is suddenly legally making decisions for you. That could be a nightmare. And I don't recommend giving someone power of attorney unless you have discussed it with him or her first. You definitely want to be confident that they understand what your wishes are and are willing to do what you are asking.

One thing to be aware of is what could happen if you give someone a general power of attorney, meaning you don't limit what decisions they can make for you, or worse yet, don't limit the circumstances when it is in effect. Someone whom has general power of attorney from you can run all of your business affairs at any time, including opening and closing bank accounts, signing contracts that bind you legally and buying and selling your possessions. That is a lot of power over your life to give anyone, so be sure to put some thought into it before you do this.

You can sometimes find pre-printed or "boilerplate" power of attorney forms at office supply stores. All you need to do with these forms is to fill in the blanks. There are also books available on how to execute several types of legal documents on your own. Check out the Internet as well for guidance and forms. Be aware that some states have specific requirements for what information needs to be included for a power of attorney to be valid. Given the complex legal nature of these forms, you may want to consult an attorney for assistance in executing them. Some HIV/AIDS service organizations are able to either assist you in executing the legal forms mentioned in this chapter or provide a referral to an attorney that will help you for free or at a reduced fee.

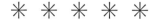

Health Care Power of Attorney and Living Will

A health care power of attorney is used to designate someone to make health care decisions on your behalf. You may see it referred to also as a medical power of attorney or health care proxy. Its most common use related to HIV is to designate someone to make health care decisions for you when you are incapacitated or otherwise unable to make them for yourself. This power covers medical treatment decisions, including whether or not to withhold such treatment. If you don't have a health care power of attorney in place, the authority to make these decisions on your behalf will usually default to your next of kin.

A living will is used to communicate your wishes to your treating physician regarding end-of-life care. This is where the common notion of "pulling the plug" comes in. If you have specific wishes about the use of life support or other life extending measures, you may want to complete a living will to legally ensure that your physician knows of your wishes and will follow them. Otherwise, your next of kin or the person named in your health care power of attorney could decide to ignore your wishes and make their own decision. You might consider executing both a health care power of attorney and living will, if having your wishes followed is important to you.

All the advice and cautions for power of attorney decisions apply to health care power of attorney decisions as well. However, whereas you might be able to undo a financial or legal transaction after you recover from your incapacity, undoing a medical decision might be much more difficult, especially if the decision was to take you off of life support! Give a lot of consideration to whom you would entrust this power. Family members might not be the best choice if they are too close to you to be objective in their decisions. Ditto for people you know are too emotional. My advice is to have a serious discussion with the person you choose, making sure they are comfortable doing this and will follow whatever your wishes are. For myself, I chose a close friend who has shown me time and time again that when it comes time to make the tough decisions, she puts her emotions aside and does whatever is necessary. Decide what qualities are important for you in this instance and choose accordingly.

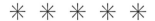

Guardianship

If you have sole legal custody of children under the age of 18, you might consider providing for guardianship of them during any periods in which you are incapacitated. Naturally, careful consideration should be given regarding who should care for and make decisions for your children when you can't. You may be relying on relatives to take care of your children during these times, but without a legal designation from you, they can't legally sign anything on the child's behalf including medical treatment releases, hospital admission forms, or even school permission slips. Unless you have addressed it in your will as discussed in the section below, you might also want to plan for guardianship for these same children in case of your death. For assistance in executing guardianship papers, you might want to consult the same resources outlined above for power of attorney.

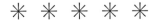

Estate Planning

I know I have been pushing you to stay present focused, but this is the one time where contemplating your own death may be beneficial to your peace of mind. If you have already executed power of attorney forms, a living will, and possibly guardianship papers, then you are in a good frame of mind to finish putting your legal affairs in order. Most people feel a sense of relief after taking care of their estate details. However, if the topic is causing you a lot of stress or discomfort, stop and breathe for a moment. If you still feel like it is too much to handle right now, then come back to this section another time when it is more comfortable for you.

A will is the legal document commonly used to express how you would like your estate to be distributed after your death. The legal requirements for a will to be valid vary from state to state. Similar to power of attorney, you might want to consider consulting an attorney or getting assistance from your local HIV/AIDS service organization. There are also many excellent kits on the market that will guide you through preparing and executing a will yourself.

In case you didn't know, you aren't legally required to execute a will. If you die without a will, your estate will be divided up according to the law in your state. Normally, these laws distribute your estate to your family, starting with your spouse and children. Executing a will generally allows you to override these laws and decide for yourself how your estate will be divided.

If you do decide to execute a will, then there are a few decisions you may want to contemplate ahead of time. First, you will have to choose an executor, meaning someone who will have the legal authority to wrap up your affairs. Second, if you have children under 18 in your sole legal custody, you may want to consider who should have custody of them, unless you want to let the court decide. If you have already asked someone to take custody after your death, putting that wish into your will makes it much more difficult for someone else to try and wrestle custody away from them. Third, make a list of any personal items that you wish to go to someone in particular. Finally, if you have specific wishes for funeral services or what should happen with your body, write them down for inclusion in your will so there is no confusion. By giving some thought to these items ahead of time, you will be sure to end up with a will that reflects your wishes and lets you have peace of mind about your affairs.

✳ ✳ ✳ ✳ ✳

Helpful Exercises

Insurance

Health, life, and disability insurance policies become valuable assets to people with HIV because they provide financial protection, affordable access to health care and security for your loved ones in case something happens to you. Which of these types of insurance do you currently have? Did you get them on your own or through your employer? Do you have any other insurance through your employer such as a long-term care policy?

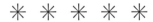

Be sure to hang on to any insurance policies you already have if you can afford the premiums. Now that you have HIV, getting an individual health, life or disability insurance policy from a regular insurance company is highly unlikely. However, you can still get these types of insurance through your employer's group policies.

Your employer may offer more than one health insurance option, causing you to wonder if you should make a switch now that you have HIV. Do you have any fears about your current insurance option? Are you afraid that you won't get the medical service that you need if you become seriously ill? Why? What are the other health insurance options available to you? Do these options offer you more freedom in choosing a doctor than your current plan? Is that freedom important to you? Why?

For each insurance option, consider looking at the following: the monthly premium cost to you, the amount that you have to pay each time that you see a doctor, any annual deductible that has to be met before you get coverage, and what the limit is on annual out-of-pocket expenses that you will have to pay. Try and balance these costs with the amount of freedom to choose your doctors, the convenience to you of the location where medical services are provided, and whether or not you can keep your current doctor. Can you fit all that in your head at one time? Good luck! Take a moment now to try and organize some of that information in your journal. You will likely have to do some research to find out some specifics about costs and coverage.

Hopefully this process helped you to reach a decision that will work for you right now. If you do choose to change your option and then find it isn't working out the way you had hoped, you can usually change it again the following year when your employer has another annual open enrollment period.

If you have left your employer recently or are thinking of doing so, you may be eligible for a COBRA extension of your insurance. To get this insurance, however, you have to pay each month 102% of the amount your employer pays to insure you. Here is an example of how this might look:

Current Health Insurance Premium Paid by You Per Month Per Month	Current Cost to Employer to Provide Health Insurance to You	Your COBRA Premium Per Month (102%)
$40	$230	$235

Shocking, yes? If you are in this situation, find out from your employer how much you would have to pay each month to keep your current health insurance. Now that you know the cost, can you afford to pay it? If you are already on COBRA and your 18 months are about to expire, have you looked into getting a HIPAA extension? Have you explored any other insurance options offered in your state or city? Check with your local HIV/AIDS service organization for the latest information on all these programs. Use your journal to make notes during your research of COBRA, HIPAA, and other federal and state insurance programs. Once you have your plan in place, don't be afraid to enlist your local HIV/AIDS organizations or other community resources to help you get enrolled in plans that you may qualify for.

Rainy Day Savings

Even though you may have a job and different types of insurance, it is still possible for life to toss you an emergency that requires you to come up with some money immediately. Do you have any money saved that you can easily access? How much? What is it invested in? How long would it take for you to get this money? What kind of interest rate is it earning?

Even if you can put away just a few dollars a week, it will add up over time. Actually, how much you save may not be as important in the end as where you put this money. It has to be placed in an account, investment, or location where you can get to it quickly and easily, hopefully in less than 24 hours. Take a moment to think about your finances and see if you have a few dollars a week to put in this fund. Start creating your plan of how much you will save each week and where you will put it. The peace of mind that comes with it is priceless.

Retirement Planning

Retirement? You may have thought that it was out of the question when you heard your diagnosis. Hopefully now you know that a long peaceful future with HIV is a possibility. Do you have any retirement savings now? How much? What types of accounts are they in? Are you continuing to add to them? How much do you add per week or month? Does your company have a pension plan? Are you relying on a governmental program like Social Security for part of your future retirement benefits?

The biggest question with retirement savings, of course, is how much is enough? I wish I could tell you, but everyone's needs are different. Because of this, it's best to get a financial advisor to help you. Your employer might offer this service to you as part of your retirement plan, so check with your plan administrator. If not, your local HIV/AIDS service organization may be able to refer you to a financial advisor who will help you for free or at a reduced fee.

Now that you have HIV, you may be concerned about putting more money in a retirement account. What are your fears in this area? Are you worried that you won't live long enough to get any benefits from this money? Or are you concerned that you might need these funds sooner than retirement and not be able to access them? Write in your journal whatever your thoughts are right now about this topic.

Money in most retirement accounts can be accessed before retirement in case of emergencies, and penalties for withdrawal are sometimes waived. Use a page in your journal to work on your retirement plan, now that you know that you may actually reach retirement age. Look at what you already have in your retirement accounts, what your financial needs might be at retirement, and how much you can spare from your current income to try and reach this goal. Makes notes from any research that you do, including information learned from phones calls you make and from any advisor you contact.

Power of Attorney

A power of attorney allows someone to take over your financial and legal affairs, excluding health care decisions. If you were unable to make decisions for yourself for a period of time, what types of decisions would you need someone to make concerning your financial and legal matters? Would you want someone to do things like pay your bills, renew your lease, or withdraw money from your bank?

Are there specific circumstances under which you would want someone making these decisions for you? Would you prefer instead to give this person this power during any period in which you are unable to make them for yourself?

Now you know what power that you would give someone and when you would give it. It's now time to consider the person or persons to whom would you give it. In your journal, make a list of the people in your life to whom you would consider giving this power. Next to each name, write the reasons why this person would be a good candidate to have your power of attorney. When you are finished, go back and choose the one person on the list who seems best for the job.

There you have your power of attorney in a nutshell. You have decided what powers to give, when they can be used and who should use them. A few more questions remain. How long do you want this document to be in effect? Consider including an expiration date in the agreement. Also, how do you know that the person you choose will follow your wishes? Talk to them about it. You can list alternates in the document in case the person that you select is unable or unwilling to act on your behalf.

You can get power of attorney forms from some office supply stores, websites, and legal form books. You may want to contact your local HIV/AIDS service organization for assistance as each state has its own requirements as to what needs to be on the form in order for it to be valid. If they can't help you, they may be able to refer you to an attorney who will assist you for free or at a reduced fee. Use your journal to takes notes during your search for assistance in completing this document. Once you have this power attorney in place, don't forget to give a copy to the person that you chose. This will save them from having to ransack your house first before they can conduct business on your behalf.

Health Care Power of Attorney and Living Will

A health care power of attorney allows someone to take over your health care decisions. It is sometimes called a health care proxy or medical power of attorney. If you were unable to make decisions for yourself for a period of time, what types of decisions would you want someone making about your health care? Would you like someone to make *any* decision that comes up in general? Is there a particular type of treatment that you do or don't want? Are there times where you would want medical treatment withheld?

Are there specific circumstances under which you would want someone making these health care decisions for you? Would you prefer instead to give them this power during any period in which you are unable to make them for yourself?

Here is a big question—to whom would you give this kind of power over your life? Make a list of people in your journal, and include next to each name the reasons why this person would be a good candidate for this role. When you are finished, go back to your list and choose the person that seems best for this responsibility.

You don't have to choose just one. You can designate alternates in case the first person you choose is unable or unwilling to make the decisions for you. The important thing to remember is that if you decide not to use a health care power of attorney and then become unable to make decisions for yourself, the power to make these types of decisions usually falls legally upon your next of kin.

When choosing someone for this role, don't forget that it is much harder to undo a medical decision than a financial or legal one. In other words, give your choice some serious thought! Definitely have a conversation with the person you choose and make certain they are ready to follow your wishes. Don't forget to consider using an expiration date to force yourself to review your arrangements periodically.

A living will is used to inform your physician legally about your end-of-care wishes. Do you have any specific wishes about the use of life support or other life extending measures? Is there some medical procedure you don't want used on you?

States have very strict requirements about what is necessary for a health care power of attorney or a living will to be valid. You can get these forms from some office supply stores, websites, and legal form books. You may want to contact your local HIV/AIDS service organization for assistance as each state has its own requirements as to what needs to be on the form for it to be valid. If they can't help you, then they may be able to refer you to an attorney who will assist you for free or at a reduced fee. Do some research about the resources available to assist you and make notes in your journal. Come up with your plan now for getting these documents in place, especially if you think that having them would bring you peace of mind.

Give a copy of your health care power of attorney to the person you've chosen to make decisions for you. This way they can immediately begin to make decisions about your health care if you become unable to make them for yourself. You may need immediate treatment to save your life. Also, be sure to give a copy of your living will to your doctor so he or she can carry out your wishes.

Guardianship

If you have sole legal custody of children under the age of 18, then consider whom you would want to care for them during times when you are unable to take care of them for health or other reasons. Make a list of those you think would be good candidates for this type of responsibility. Next to each name, write the reasons why this person would be a good choice.

When you are finished, pick the person on your list that appears to be the best fit for this serious responsibility.

When creating guardianship papers, it's important to remember either to include an expiration date or to review the document periodically to avoid giving temporary custody of your children to someone that you no longer wish to have it. Use all the resources mentioned above for power of attorney to help you in executing these papers. Each state has its own requirements for guardianship papers to be valid, so consider seeking out some legal guidance. As always, give a copy of the executed papers to the person you chose to have temporary custody of your children. Use your journal to record notes during your research and create your plan of action that ensures your children are taken care of.

Estate Planning

Thinking about your death is probably something you've done too much of in the recent past. Most people, however, feel a sense of relief once they have their estate affairs in order. Do you have a will already? If so, when was the last time you updated it? Does it still reflect your current wishes? If you don't have a will, why not? What has stopped you from executing one in the past?

The requirements for executing a valid will vary widely from state to state. You should definitely consider seeking legal assistance from your local HIV/AIDS service organization or an attorney. However, there are some basic decisions that need to be made in any will, so let's discuss them to help you prepare. The first one is choosing an executor. The executor is responsible for making sure the will is followed and the business aspects of your estate are wrapped up. They will pull together your assets, settle your accounts, and distribute your estate according to your wishes. They are also responsible for filing income tax returns for your estate. Who would be a good choice to be your executor? For each candidate you identify in your journal, give the reasons why you think that person would make a good executor for your estate.

You can also name alternate executors in case the person you chose is unable or unwilling to serve as your executor. The second thing to consider is the legal custody of your children under the age of 18, if you have any. You may have already executed guardianship papers for when you are incapacitated during life. However, after you have died, the court will decide who gets custody of your children if you had sole legal custody of them and haven't made your wishes known legally. You might do this by including these wishes in your will or by executing a guardianship document that covers custody after your death. Consider seeking legal assistance and guidance as to what works best in your state. Use your journal now to record your thoughts and feelings regarding the best person to have custody of your children after you die. Is your choice the same person you named in your guardianship papers for temporary custody? If not, why not? Who is a better choice? Why?

Next, you may have prized possessions that you want specific people to have. Maybe they are family heirlooms or sentimental reminders of events in the past. Think for a moment, and then make a list of these items and who you might want to have them. If you can't decide exactly who should get an item, list more than one name if it helps.

Rather than giving a certain possession, you may want to give a dollar amount to specific people instead. You could specify an exact dollar amount, or you could state a percentage, like 30% of your remaining estate. Keep in mind that creditors get paid first, so any gifts you make might be reduced or eliminated if there is not enough money left in your estate to pay them. Use your journal now to identify the people you would want to receive some money from your estate. Next to each name, you might want to specify dollar amounts or percentages as a general guideline so you will be ready when you execute your will. Also, if there are people in your life you want to get nothing from your estate, you may want to include that fact in your will so that it is clear that you meant to exclude them rather than just forgot about them. This may save your heirs from having to deal with someone contesting your will.

Finally, you may want to include any wishes you have regarding your final arrangements. Do you want a funeral, memorial service, or nothing at all? Do you want to be buried or cremated? If cremated, do you want someone in particular to have your ashes? Do you want your ashes spread somewhere specific?

Great! Now you have an idea of what you might want to put into your will. As I mentioned, your local HIV/AIDS service organization may be able to give you assistance with executing your will or make a referral to a local attorney that will do it for free or at a reduced fee. Also, there are books and software programs out there designed to help you execute a will on your own. Use your journal now to make notes during your research and begin formulating your plan for getting a will in place. Be sure to give a copy of your completed will to your executor. And keep a copy in a safe place for yourself.

Chapter 6 Checklist

Complete the following checklist in your journal. Putting your financial and legal matters in order will give you the peace of mind to focus on the next stage in your journey. Chapter 6 ends your current stage, *Managing Your Details.* **DO NOT** continue on to the next stage in Chapter 7 until you have accomplished every item on the checklists in Chapters 1 through 6. Number a page in your journal from 1 to 50, then record the date that you accomplish each step below.

Insurance

1. Identified what types of insurance you already have and whether they are individual or employer group policies

2. Accepted that you probably won't be able to get certain types of insurance on your own now that you have HIV

3. Acknowledged your concerns about your current health insurance option through your employer and whether you might want to change it

4. Analyzed the potential costs of changing your health insurance option and weighed this cost against factors like freedom of choice and convenience

5. Decided whether or not to change your health insurance option, recognizing that you may be able to change it again in a year

6. Determined whether or not your life or disability insurance provided by your employer ends when you leave your job or can be continued afterwards

7. Recognized that the federal laws COBRA and HIPAA may allow you to keep your health insurance indefinitely if you pay the monthly premium

8. Contacted your local HIV/AIDS organization for more information about federal, state, and local insurance programs and assistance in filing any claims.

Rainy Day Savings

9. Identified if you have any funds you could access quickly and easily and the amount of these funds

10. Acknowledged there may be emergencies that require you to come up with money quickly to avoid panic and stress

11. Realized that even a small amount of money saved each week will add up over time

12. Accepted that your rainy day savings should be invested in something stable that is easy to access like a savings or money market account, and not in time deposits, stocks, or other investments that need to be sold before you can get the funds

13. Created and began to follow a plan for building a rainy day fund, if you can afford it, to find the peace of mind that is priceless

Retirement Planning

14. Identified what retirement savings you have, what types of accounts they are in, and how much you are adding to them each month

15. Realized that you can still access your retirement savings for emergency cash through loans or withdrawals, depending upon the type of account

16. Contacted the plan administrator of your 401(k) or other type of employer retirement account to find out about ways to get cash from your account if needed

17. Recognized that you will have to pay incomes taxes and possibly penalties on any withdrawals that you make

18. Contacted your employer or your local HIV/AIDS service organization for assistance with retirement planning or referral to a financial advisor that will help you possibly for free or at a reduced price

19. Began to organize and create a retirement plan to ensure your future needs are met

Power of Attorney

20. Identified what financial and legal decisions you would
    need made during periods in which you can't make
    them for yourself
21. Identified what events or circumstances would trigger
    a period where someone else made decisions for you
22. Identified to whom you would give this power during
    these periods and the reasons why you would want to
    give it to them
23. Discussed your wishes with the person you choose,
    making sure they are comfortable with doing this
    for you
24. Remembered to consider adding an expiration date to
    avoid having someone that you no longer trust making
    your decisions
25. Contacted your local HIV/AIDS service organization
    for assistance in completing this document and possi-
    ble referral to an attorney to help you for free or at a
    reduced price
26. Remembered to give a copy of the executed document
    to the person you chose to act on your behalf

Health Care Power of Attorney and Living Will

27. Identified what health care decisions you would need
    made during periods in which you can't make them
    for yourself
28. Identified what events or circumstances would trigger
    a period where someone else made decisions for you
29. Identified to whom you would give this power during
    these periods and the reasons why you would want to
    give it to them
30. Discussed your wishes with the person you chose, mak-
    ing sure they are comfortable with doing this for you
31. Remembered to consider adding an expiration date to
    avoid having someone you no longer trust making
    your decisions

32. Recognized that this health care decision making ability will likely default legally to your next of kin during these periods if you don't execute this form
33. Considered executing a living will if you have end-of-cares wishes, such as not being put on life support
34. Contacted your local HIV/AIDS service organization for assistance in completing these documents and possible referral to an attorney to help you for free or at a reduced price
35. Remembered to give a copy of the executed documents to the person you chose to act on your behalf as well as to your physician

Guardianship

36. Determined whether you have sole legal custody of a child under 18, not just visitation rights
37. Identified who you would like to take care of your children during any periods you can't, along with the reasons why you chose this person
38. Discussed your wishes with the person that you chose, making sure they are comfortable with doing this for you
39. Contacted your local HIV/AIDS service organization for assistance in completing these papers and possible referral to an attorney to help you for free or at a reduced price
40. Remembered to give a copy of the executed document to the person that you chose to have temporary custody of your children during these times

Estate Planning

41. Acknowledged your feelings and fears about considering your own death and decided whether or not you should continue planning right now
42. Considered consulting a financial or tax advisor if your estate is large or complicated

43. Recognized that a will is not legally required and that your estate would likely go to your family if you died with no will

44. Identified who you would like to be your executor and the reasons why you chose this person

45. Identified who you would want to have custody of your minor children after your death, including why you chose this person

46. Determined if you want certain people to get specific items

47. Determined if you want to give a certain amount of cash or a percentage of the estate to specific people

48. Determined if you have any wishes about your final arrangements, including type of service conducted, if any, and disposition of your body or ashes.

49. Contacted your local HIV/AIDS service organization for assistance in completing this document and possible referral to an attorney to help you for free or at a reduced price

50. Remembered to give a copy of the executed document to the person that you chose to be your executor

Resource Examples

Be Prepared: The Complete Financial, Legal, and Practical Guide for Living With a Life-Challenging Condition, David S. Landay

Power of Attorney Handbook, Edward A. Haman

Nolo's Simple Will Book, Denis Clifford

The Complete Idiot's Guide® to Wills and Estate, Stephen M. Maple and Chris Eliopoulos

How to Write Your Own Living Will, Edward A. Haman and Douglas E. Godbe

Nolo Press, www.nolopress.com
Look for: Do-it-yourself guidance and forms for legal issues, including wills, power of attorney, and health care power of attorney

Lambda Legal Defense and Education Fund,
www.lambdalegal.org
Look for: Guidance on completing legal forms along with referral to a local attorney to assist you

Partnership for Caring, www.partnershipforcaring.org
Look for: Free download of medical power of attorney and living will forms for each state

Health Insurance InfoNet, www.healthinsuranceinfo.net
Look for: Guide for each state on how to get and keep health insurance, including information on your legal protections, COBRA and state insurance programs

U.S. Dept. of Labor, Employee Benefits Security Administration, www.dol.gov/dol/ebsa
Look for: Guidance on and handling of complaints about COBRA, HIPAA and pension rights

Chapter 7

Healing the Mind, Body and Spirit

Crisis ended? Check. Foundation built? Check. HIV incorporated into daily life? Check. Hmm, you have done everything you were supposed to do so far. Why isn't that peace with HIV here yet? What more could be left? I am glad you asked. *Achieving Your Balance* is your last stage.

To achieve the lasting peace with HIV, you will need first to find the balance in your life. When the mind, body, and spirit work in balance and harmony within you, vibrant health and vitality is the result. You achieve a sense of balance, well-being, and contentment. When one of these areas goes out of balance, however, you will experience discomfort in the other two areas as well.

For example, your mind was working overtime during your crisis period, imagining all sorts of awful stuff for the future. At the same time, I bet that your body was tight, tired, or achy. You probably also felt depressed, disheartened, or hopeless. See the link? It stands to reason that to return to a state of vibrant health and peace, healing needs to occur in your mind, in your body, and in your spirit. This is the basic philosophy of holistic medical approaches, in which the goal is to treat the source of the *dis*-ease, not just the symptoms. Only when the source is addressed and removed can the mind, body, and spirit return to their balanced state, restoring the vibrant health that we are trying to achieve each day.

Achieving this balance may sound simple enough, but how do you get there? You are a lot closer than you might think.

You have already done a lot of work on your mind by being present focused, and learning how to relax through breathing and through meditating. Your new healthy habits should be doing a great job of supporting your body. Now in this final stage, let's discuss some ways to enliven and strengthen your spirit. As you develop your spirit, you can also explore using some holistic methods discussed below to bring these three areas into balance. Once that balance is yours, living in peace with HIV is certain to follow sooner rather than later. Guaranteed.

Explore Your Spirituality

Let me make a quick distinction between spirituality and religion before some of you tune out like I used to do when someone mentioned those two words to me. Spirituality is an individual pursuit whereas religion is a group activity. Spirituality is about looking inside yourself to discover who you are, what you believe, and what you are here to do. It is all about you. Religion is when people come together to celebrate their spirituality as a group. Some religions have a detailed comprehensive set of beliefs that all members are assumed to accept and personify in living their lives. Catholicism is an example of this type of religion. Some religions have more general beliefs that members can accept or reject without concern. Religious Science is a good example of this approach. There are many more aspects to religion for you to explore, but I hope that my brief description has helped you to understand the distinction between it and spirituality, in case you were unsure.

No doubt at some point since your diagnosis, you have questioned what the meaning of life is or why you are even here if something like this is going to happen to you. Who can answer those questions? Maybe you. If not today, perhaps someday. Exploring your spirituality doesn't have to be a formal or complex pursuit. It can take whatever form you are comfortable with. Just keep in mind a popular adage—change your thinking, change your life. For years, my method of exploring my spirituality was very solitary, buying and reading books on a variety of topics that I thought would assist me in developing my self awareness. Over the past two years, I have decided to explore the sense of community associated with religion by attending a few services and talking with other people. Hearing about other people's journeys has helped me to learn more about myself in some ways. As always, do whatever might be comfortable for you.

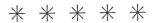

Do Some Volunteer Work

I have come to believe that doing volunteer work is the single best activity that you can do to heal your spirit. The reason is simple—doing it takes you out of your head and into your heart. When you are helping people in need, you are opening your heart and bringing alive that part of you that feels connected to other people. This feeling is priceless, especially in those moments where you feel alone in the world. That connection helps you to know that it is not true.

You're likely to gain some valuable perspective from this experience. Chances are, you'll encounter people who are worse off than you are, and this alone may help you to feel better about your situation in some small way. Taking it one step further, if you are able to open your heart and find a way to help make that person's life a little bit better, even just for a moment, you may find that the healing effect on your spirit is beyond anything you could possibly have imagined. Maybe all it takes is a kind word or a smile. Consider giving it a try.

In trying to choose where to spend your time, don't feel any pressure to focus your attention on HIV/AIDS service organizations. Definitely, if you are drawn to help those people in need because of HIV/AIDS, then put your efforts there. But if you still feel like you couldn't stop yourself from internalizing other people's experiences with HIV, you should probably avoid this type of work for the time being. There are so many other organizations out there that serve the needs of your community, many of which count people with HIV among their clients. I choose to split my time between a HIV-related charity and a general community one. It keeps me grounded and allows my spirit to stay in harmony.

✳ ✳ ✳ ✳ ✳

Bring Your Inner Child Out to Play

There is nothing that enlivens your spirit more than having a little fun. You've probably spent a tremendous amount of time being serious ever since your diagnosis, especially in light of the hefty decisions you've had to make. Now that you are healing, consider having spontaneous moments of playful joy.

Sing along with a television commercial or the theme song of your favorite show. Make goofy faces in the mirror or tell some silly jokes to a friend. Draw stick figures or colorful doodles on the envelopes of your monthly bills before you send them. Hey, you could try my favorite thing—push your shopping cart at the store, then lean up against it and ride it until it stops. Then do it again. Just don't run anyone over or destroy a display of canned peas! A friend recently told me that I look like a little kid when I ride on the cart. Exactly. He should have seen me the time that I jumped up on top and pretended to be swimming.

Society has taught us that as mature adults, we should be serious and responsible. Okay, but not every waking moment. We were all experts at being playful when we were kids. Personally, I don't think we've lost that part of us, but rather we have chosen not to acknowledge it very often. Try and remember how much fun it was to take a mundane task and make it into a little game. If you are afraid of what others may think of your childlike behavior, then just do it when you're alone. Regardless of what form it takes, it is guaranteed to lift your spirits and make you smile, at least for a moment. That is definitely a good start.

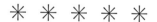

Consider Holistic Therapy

If you were having a serious problem with your eyes, you would go see a specialist for treatment to correct the problem. You would want someone helping you who really understood your condition and how to treat it. Along the same lines, if you need help in balancing your mind, body, and spirit, you might consider going to see a holistic practitioner. Holistic medicine is designed to address the *dis*-ease in your life that may be causing this imbalance.

Energy is what flows through you, connecting your mind, body, and spirit. Holistic practitioners are people with a gift for sensing energy within your body. Their skills also extend to helping you remove energy blocks within yourself. Holistic practitioners use a variety of therapies called modalities, including acupressure, acupuncture, hot stones, energy balancing, healing touch, reiki, shamanic counseling, chiropractic adjustments, massage, foot reflexology, and herbal treatments. Once the energy is flowing freely again between your mind, body and spirit, the balance between them is restored and your goal of living in peace with HIV back on track.

There are some HIV/AIDS service organizations dedicated specifically to helping you access these holistic therapies for free or at a reduced cost. This is possible because local holistic practitioners have donated their time and talents out of a desire to help people with HIV heal. My former chiropractor generously sees people with HIV for free and swears he has helped some people double their T-cells through his therapy. You never know. That could be true. All medical claims aside, I have tried many of these holistic therapies and found them to have beneficial effects for me. Even if I don't sense an immediate change in my energy after a treatment, I am definitely more relaxed and peaceful at the end. This kind of peace is exactly what you are trying to achieve in your experience with HIV. You might find holistic therapy is a good way for you to get there.

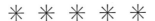

Helpful Exercises

To begin, let's try to form a picture of how you are doing right now. Do you feel as though your mind, body, and spirit are in balance at this moment? If not, what do you think is the source of the imbalance or discomfort? How is it showing up in your mind, your body, and your spirit?

Explore Your Spirituality

Spirituality is all about you. It is what you believe about yourself, the world, and life. When you hear the word spirituality, what do you think of? What is your spirituality like? Do you have any particular beliefs that you embrace?

Spirituality is often confused with religion. Spirituality is an individual pursuit while religion is a group activity in which people celebrate their spirituality together. Finding out who you are and why you are here might be two things that come out of your spiritual practices. Have you explored your spirituality? What methods did you use? What insights did you have about yourself, other people or life in general? Are there other ways to explore your spirituality that you would like to try?

I'll admit that I may be pushing the spirituality aspect a bit hard here. That is strange behavior for someone like me who grew up void of spirituality or religion. But to achieve that balance between mind, body, and spirit, you will need to develop your spiritual muscles. It took me almost four years of living with HIV to realize this. I hope that someday soon that you are able to do the same, and much more quickly than I did.

Use your journal now to create a plan for you to explore your spirituality and achieve the peace that comes with balance.

Do Some Volunteer Work

I think that doing volunteer work is the single best activity for enlivening your spirit. That is because volunteer work takes you out of your head and into your heart, where your spirit is. You are opening your heart to people in an effort to make their lives just a little bit better. Have you done volunteer work before? Do you do it now? What did you do and how did you feel when you did it? Do you have any fears about doing volunteer work? What are they?

You will be amazed at how much doing volunteer work does for your spirit. This work will also help you feel connected to those around you, which might lead you to remember that you are never truly alone.

So what have you decided about volunteer work? Whom would you like to help? How much time do you have to give? Jot down your ideas in your journal about how and when to give your time. Check your weekly schedule back in Chapter 3 and consider scheduling some time on it for volunteer work.

Bring Your Inner Child Out to Play

Have you spent a lot of time being serious ever since you got your diagnosis? When is the last time that you had fun? I am not talking about the fun that you planned a week in advance with your friends. I am talking about the kind of fun that happens on the spur of the moment while you were busy doing something else. What is your idea of fun? When did you last do something spontaneously fun? When is the last time that you laughed out loud at something?

As a kid, you were an expert at turning mundane tasks into a game to make them more fun. Sure, now you are a mature, responsible adult. But even mature, responsible adults have room for a little spontaneous joy. Here is my challenge to you: create a list in your journal of mundane or routine tasks that you do, and then come up with an idea of how you can make each one of them fun. After you do this, think up other ways to have a moment of fun while you are busy doing something else, like singing along loudly with the radio while you're driving or trying to catch a butterfly as you walk down the sidewalk. Use your journal to come up with your plan to drop your cares for a while and just enjoy being alive.

All right, now you are in the right frame of mind. You will be amazed at how good it feels to just cut loose for a moment and enjoy yourself. If you are too worried about what other people think to let yourself have fun in public, then do things only when you are alone so that the worry doesn't stop you. When you are smiling and laughing, it will seem like peace is just around the corner. It is.

Consider Holistic Therapy

Review what you wrote about your mind, body, and spirit at the beginning of this chapter. Recall any problems and how their symptoms were playing out in these three areas. When you hear or see the word *holistic*, what do you think of? What do you think holistic therapy is? What do you think a holistic practitioner does? How could they help you with your problem?

Holistic practitioners are specialists at sensing energy within your body. To help you to remove any energy blocks, they use a variety of treatment methods. Below is a partial list of modalities with descriptions. Note in your journal any that sound interesting to you. Don't forget to research other holistic treatments not listed here and make notes to follow up on them later.

Acupressure is a massage technique from Chinese medicine that focuses on the body's pressure points and meridians. It is used to treat pain of all sorts including muscular pain, headache, and mental stress.

Acupuncture is a Chinese medical practice that involves inserting thin needles at specified points on the body to manipulate the flow of energy. It is used to treat a variety of symptoms, including peripheral neuropathy. It is also used to enhance overall health and promote relaxation.

Biofeedback is a stress-management technique used to reduce the occurrence of stress-related disorders.

Chiropractic treatments involve the manipulation of the body to correct defective alignments of the neck, back and extremities. Treatments are administered by a licensed Doctor of Chiropractic and are used to ease nerve impairment and pain.

Cranial sacral work is a massage technique that uses light touch to focus on the nervous system to reduce stress and encourage natural healing.

Hatha yoga is a form of exercise for the body, mind, and spirit that combines deep breathing and concentration with gentle movement to build posture, balance, flexibility, and strength.

Massage therapy uses a variety of techniques, from deep tissue to light touch. Treatments are used to relax the connective tissues to enhance blood and lymph circulation and to relieve stress.

Reflexology is an ancient form of massage therapy that works on the reflex points located on the hands and feet. Its benefits include improving blood circulation and well-being, stress relief, and maintaining a healthy balance between mind and body.

Reiki is a form of hands-on touch that guides life-force energy for stress reduction and natural healing of the mind, body, and spirit.

Shiatsu is a form of energy work using the application of thumbs, elbows, or knees along the body's meridian lines and pressure points. It is used to restore energy imbalances within the body.

There are some HIV/AIDS service organizations dedicated specifically to bringing these services to HIV-positive people. Check with your local HIV/AIDS service organization to see if they have some of these services or can refer you to local practitioners who will see you for free or at a reduced price. Some of these services may be covered by your health insurance, so you might try calling your plan administrator to get names of practitioners near you. Your doctor may know of some of these practitioners as well. You can also try searching online using such keywords as *holistic* along with your city or state name or the name of the treatment that you would like to receive. Use your journal to make notes during your search and to create your plan for balance and wellness. Once you have the energy flowing freely again between your mind, body, and spirit, you will be a lot closer to the peace with HIV that you've been working towards.

Chapter 7 Checklist

Now that you have finished your exercises, complete the following checklist in your journal. Number a page in your journal from 1 to 22, and note the date that you complete each step below. Once you have accomplished every item on this list, you will have completed the final stage of your journey towards living in peace with HIV. Congratulations on all your hard work!

First Step:

1. Acknowledged whether your mind, body, and spirit are currently in balance, and if not, what the symptoms and the source of the problem are

Explore Your Spirituality

2. Acknowledged what spirituality means to you, what your spirituality is like, and any particular beliefs that you may have
3. Recognized the difference between spirituality and religion
4. Identified ways in which you have explored your spirituality and what you learned from using each method
5. Realized that developing your spiritual muscles is necessary to strike a balance between mind, body, and spirit
6. Created and began to follow a plan to explore your spirituality and achieve the peace that comes with balance

Do Some Volunteer Work

7. Acknowledged your feelings (and fears) about doing volunteer work, if you have done any in the past and how you felt doing it
8. Recognized that doing volunteer work can help enliven your spirit by having you open up your heart to help others
9. Realized that doing volunteer work may help you to gain perspective on your situation as you see others who need more help than you do
10. Acknowledged that you don't have to limit your volunteer work to just organizations that serve people with HIV/AIDS
11. Created and began to follow a plan to do some volunteer work to help develop your spirituality
12. Put time for volunteer work on the weekly schedule that you created in Chapter 3

Bring Your Inner Child Out to Play

13. Acknowledged what your idea of fun is and when you last did something fun or spontaneous
14. Identified mundane or routine tasks that you do and how you could make them into a game or at least more fun

15. Imagined other ways you could have fun at any moment when doing things like driving, shopping, or walking down the sidewalk
16. Recognized that you could have these fun moments alone if you are concerned about other people seeing you

Consider Holistic Therapy

17. Identified what you think holistic therapy is and how it may help you with the problem and symptoms you identified at the beginning of this chapter
18. Realized that holistic medicine attempts to correct the *dis*-ease in your life by addressing the symptoms and removing the cause
19. Reviewed the holistic therapy checklist and identified ones in which you might be interested, understanding that there are more therapies than what is on the list
20. Contacted your local HIV/AIDS service organization, health insurance company, or doctor to assist you in locating these services in your area
21. Realized that your local HIV/AIDS service organization might be able to arrange for you to have these services for free or at a reduced price
22. Created and began to follow a plan to use holistic therapies to help restore and maintain the balance between your mind, body, and spirit

Resource Examples

Anatomy of the Spirit, Carol Myss

Your Body Believes Every Word that You Say, Barbara Hoberman Levine

Smile for No Good Reason, Lee L. Jampolsky

Manifesto for a New Medicine: Your Guide to Healing Partnerships and the Wise Use of Alternative Therapies, James Samuel Gordon

You Can Heal Your Life, Louise L. Hay

New Healing Herbs: The Classic Guide to Nature's Best Medicine, Michael Castleman

Resilient Spirit: Transforming Suffering into Insight and Renewal, Polly Young-Eisendrath

Creative Visualization, Shakti Gawain

The Power of Your Subconscious Mind, Joseph Murphy, et al

Buddhist AIDS Project, www.buddhistaidsproject.org
Look for: Buddhist philosophy to helping you learn to live with HIV/AIDS

By Region Network, www.byregion.net
Look for: Global listings of local healers and holistic practitioners by region

The Body Positive, www.thebody.com
Look for: Quality of life articles discussing use of holistic therapy in improving health

HIV Wellness Center, www.main.org/hivwell
Look for: Detailed descriptions of many holistic therapies

Living Now, www.livingnow.com.au
Look for: Articles and stories supporting the integration of mind, body and soul in all areas of life

Council of Religious AIDS Networks, www.aidsfaith.org
Look for: Discussions about aspects of AIDS and religion

Conclusion

Keeping the Peace

Congratulations on completing your journey! To celebrate your success, take a moment and reflect upon how far that you have come in the time since you started reading this book and creating your journal. Remember what you were thinking about your future as you read the first page. Reread any thoughts or notes that you wrote to yourself in your journal early on in this process. Maybe some of these thoughts seem far removed from you now, or perhaps they are still there but not affecting you as much or in the same way. Either way, you are now able to enjoy your life in this moment, without worry for the future destroying your happiness.

So have you found your peace with HIV yet? I am guessing you have but may not know it. You are probably thinking you haven't found it because you aren't completely comfortable with every aspect having the disease. Who is? Everyone has areas of living with HIV with which they are less comfortable—mine is dating. All this means is that you will focus some extra attention on these areas as they surface in your daily life. I bet if you think back to before you were diagnosed, you will realize you already had areas of your life with which you weren't completely comfortable. So maybe not that much is different now in this respect.

Don't overlook the fact that the peace with HIV you have achieved has come from becoming more present focused, more centered, and more balanced in your mind, body, and spirit. With a solid foundation like that, it doesn't matter what life throws at you, HIV-related or not. You will be able to work through any situation or feeling which surfaces without it taking a major toll on your mental health and overall well-being. I know this firsthand from my experience of writing this book.

To give you meaningful guidance, I have shared many important moments from my journey with HIV, some of which were the most traumatic, emotional experiences of my life. When reliving these moments in my head, I surprised myself with the level of peace and contentment I felt instead of the emotional trauma that I remembered. My calm approach allowed me to finally understand what had happened to me in those moments, and even better, what I had learned from those experiences. You have this same ability now. You have worked hard to gain these skills, and while they may never be perfect, they will help you to keep the peace in your life.

By using these newfound skills, you will soon recognize that integrating HIV peacefully into your life is a sure recipe for happiness while meeting it with resistance is an invitation for a troubled existence. Go with the peace.

About The Author

Timothy J. Critzer has earned a Bachelors of Business Administration/Accounting degree from Kent State University, and a Juris Doctorate from Golden Gate University School of Law, specializing in labor, employment and public interest law. He has also achieved the designation of Certified Employee Benefits Specialist (CEBS).

Timothy has been HIV-positive since 1998 and is passionately committed to helping other HIV-positive find their peace with this condition. In addition to being a guest speaker at HIV/AIDS organizations across the country, he has also continued to support this community and to create resources for it through publishing books, developing workshops and authoring an advice column on living well with HIV and AIDS.

How to Purchase
Additional Copies

Individual Sales (for personal use)

Single copies can be purchased at:

Your local bookstore,
Amazon.com and other online retailers, or
Firsthand Books, by mail order
($16.95 plus $2.00 shipping and handling for each
copy, checks or money orders only, to the address
below)

Retail/Institutional Sales (for resale/distribution)

Special discounts are available for retailers,
wholesalers, nonprofits, governmental agencies and
other types of HIV/AIDS service organizations.

Please visit *www.firsthandbooks.com* for more details,
or call toll free (877) 582-4928. Updated contact
information and current promotions for Firsthand
Books will always be available on its website.

Volume Discounts available for all sales of 100+ books

Firsthand Books
584 Castro Street #342
San Francisco, CA 94114